T0054037

Trigger Point Therapy Made Simple

Trigger Point Therapy

MADE SIMPLE

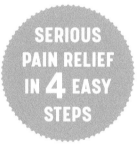

SERIOUS PAIN RELIEF IN **4** EASY STEPS

Richard Finn, LMT, CMTPT

Illustrations by Charlie Layton

ROCKRIDGE PRESS

Copyright © 2020 by Rockridge Press, Emeryville, California

No part of this publication may be reproduced, stored in a retrieval system, or transmitted in any form or by any means, electronic, mechanical, photocopying, recording, scanning, or otherwise, except as permitted under Sections 107 or 108 of the 1976 United States Copyright Act, without the prior written permission of the Publisher. Requests to the Publisher for permission should be addressed to the Permissions Department, Rockridge Press, 6005 Shellmound Street, Suite 175, Emeryville, CA 94608.

Limit of Liability/Disclaimer of Warranty: The Publisher and the author make no representations or warranties with respect to the accuracy or completeness of the contents of this work and specifically disclaim all warranties, including without limitation warranties of fitness for a particular purpose. No warranty may be created or extended by sales or promotional materials. The advice and strategies contained herein may not be suitable for every situation. This work is sold with the understanding that the Publisher is not engaged in rendering medical, legal, or other professional advice or services. If professional assistance is required, the services of a competent professional person should be sought. Neither the Publisher nor the author shall be liable for damages arising herefrom. The fact that an individual, organization, or website is referred to in this work as a citation and/or potential source of further information does not mean that the author or the Publisher endorses the information the individual, organization, or website may provide or recommendations they/it may make. Further, readers should be aware that websites listed in this work may have changed or disappeared between when this work was written and when it is read.

For general information on our other products and services or to obtain technical support, please contact our Customer Care Department within the United States at (866) 744-2665, or outside the United States at (510) 253-0500.

Rockridge Press publishes its books in a variety of electronic and print formats. Some content that appears in print may not be available in electronic books, and vice versa.

TRADEMARKS: Rockridge Press and the Rockridge Press logo are trademarks or registered trademarks of Callisto Media Inc. and/or its affiliates, in the United States and other countries, and may not be used without written permission. All other trademarks are the property of their respective owners. Rockridge Press is not associated with any product or vendor mentioned in this book.

Interior and Cover Designer: Erik Jacobsen
Art Producer: Sara Feinstein
Editor: Lauren O'Neal
Illustrations by Charlie Layton
ISBN: 978-1-64611-562-4 | eBook: 978-1-64611-563-1

R0

To my beloved bride, Carol. She has been my constant companion and helpmeet over the course of the last 35 years. She has given me comfort, a kick in the pants, or just jumped in to help in a multitude of projects— and made sure I was well loved.

Contents

Chapter Five: Arms and Hands 77

Introduction

It's 3:00 a.m., and Sally is tossing and turning. Her back pain is so severe that she can't sleep. There is no doctor or therapist awake to help her, and medication doesn't seem to make much difference. She lies in bed, suffering, as the peacefully sleeping figure beside her snores loudly. What is Sally to do?

Perhaps you've felt like Sally. Nothing is so irritating as the loneliness of pain with no hope of help. The purpose of this book is to give you that hope as well as teach you the skills and techniques you need to get relief from your pain. And there is so much you can do!

For some of you, this may be the first step on your journey toward pain relief. Others have been chipping away at this goal for some time. Wherever you are on this road, you will find material in this book to speed you on your way. You'll find foundational material along with new ideas, all of which are designed to give you important tools for this task.

My journey began when I was hit by a car while riding my bike. Years of pain ensued, followed by years of learning what helped and why. There were a lot of twists and turns that I made on my journey to relief. I've been drugged, injected, and poked by some of the best. Along the way, I became a myofascial trigger point therapist, an educator in the field, and an author. I've taught health care professionals across many disciplines and have appeared in print as well as TV and radio. Simply stated: I've probably felt your pain. I've also probably successfully treated it.

Many people seek out professional help in order to deal with their pain. Sometimes, seeing a few different types of professionals is part of the journey (especially when it comes to making sure that your pain is not actually being caused by a serious ailment). But it's also true that there's just no substitute for jumping into your own health care treatment. It's your participation that yields the greatest success. I've been there, and in this book, I'll show you what has worked for me and for many others who have followed the methods I've outlined. This book focuses on what is practical—methods that actually work. You can face your pain, understand it, and deal with it. Now you have a fighting chance. Go for it!

PART ONE

What to Know

THE FIRST PART OF THIS BOOK IS CALLED
"What to Know" because it will help you understand where your pain comes from and what you can do about it. It will lay the foundation that you need in order to understand and apply the methods detailed in part 2. Don't skip ahead because you're eager to just get started. Think of part 1 as the vocabulary for a new language—you need to understand it before you can move on to more complex concepts (like those laid out in part 2).

CHAPTER ONE

Trigger Points 101

What are trigger points? How do you get them? And how can something so small cause so much pain? This chapter will give you essential information about trigger points and trigger point therapy so you can learn about the source of your pain and how the techniques in this book can make a huge difference.

Trigger Points: The Basics

At its most basic, a trigger point is just a tender spot or knot in a muscle. That's it! Now you know as much as a lot of people. But in order to use the techniques featured in this book, you'll need to know a little more than that. So let's take a closer look at how trigger points develop and how they cause pain.

What Are Trigger Points?

To get a little more technical, a trigger point is thought to be an area where the parts of the muscle that contract have shortened. Our muscle fibers shorten and lengthen all the time as we move around, but they shouldn't stay shortened permanently. With trigger points, the shortening seems to happen right below the nerve that supplies the muscle with the signal to shorten. It's not shortened anywhere else—in fact, on either side of the knot, the fibers of the muscle are actually stretched because of the severe shortening in the middle.

This makes finding those spots easy for professionals like me. I rub my fingers over the muscle fiber or squeeze it between my fingers, looking for the tautness of the band of stretched, shortened muscle. Then I move my fingers along the band, and wham! A knot, or "nodule," is waiting for me to press it!

Those nodules cause myofascial pain, which is pain related to the muscles or fasciae (the connective tissue that covers the muscles). For a long time, science didn't understand precisely why trigger points are so tender. We finally got a better idea in 2008, when Jay Shah, a doctor at the National Institutes of Health, performed a microdialysis of the inside of a trigger point—that is to say, he analyzed fluid taken from the center of several trigger points. There he found a number of chemicals that are known to be involved in inflammation, which helps to explain why the spot is so tender.

What Causes Trigger Points?

What causes trigger points? It's a really good question, and one we can't yet fully answer. Trigger points have not been a topic of much research, because even though muscles make up half of our body weight, there isn't a medical specialty that specializes in just muscles (the way, say, a dermatologist specializes in skin or an otolaryngologist specializes in the ear, nose, and throat). In fact, the pioneering trigger point researcher David G. Simons called muscle the "orphan organ."

Additionally, trigger point nodules don't show up on standard imaging tests like CT scans, MRIs, or X-rays, because they're tiny and made of soft tissue. While blood tests can sometimes detect conditions that *accompany* trigger points, like rheumatoid arthritis, they don't give us any information about the nodules themselves.

Still, we know a bit about why our bodies create trigger points. The current thinking is that when a nerve gets irritated, it can cause the center of the muscle to shorten into a knot. That area of irritation often sends signals to other parts of the body, causing pain as well as sensations like numbness and tingling. Locating your tender spots is often the best test, and you can feel for them yourself—they can feel like a BB, a bean, or even a marble.

Trigger points often seem to develop after a physical trauma like a car accident or fall. General stress also seems to be a big factor in causing and exacerbating pain, and people with chronic diseases often develop trigger points in their muscles as well.

> Note: *Not all pain felt in muscles is related to trigger points— it can have many other causes, including ulcers, appendicitis, or renal disease. Because of this, it's important to consult with a doctor about your pain and rule out other underlying causes. If your pain has another cause, you'll need a different treatment.*

What Are the Effects of Trigger Points?

People with trigger points describe how they make them feel in a wide variety of ways. Some describe them as painful, while others report sensations like numbness and tingling. Usually the pain from a trigger point is described as "dull" and "aching." It's important to note that pain is actually an experience rather than a sensation. Your understanding of and feelings about the issue, as well as the actual physical input, determines whether your brain will output pain. Many people don't like the word "pain" but struggle to find another way to describe the sensation they feel from a trigger point.

Trigger points are often the culprit behind or a factor in other physical problems. They're common among people with fibromyalgia, arthritis, carpal tunnel syndrome, temporomandibular joint (TMJ) disorder, headaches, and plantar fasciitis, to name only a few conditions. If you have any kind of myofascial pain, it is quite likely that trigger points are part of the problem.

Because our muscles, fasciae, and nerves are all interconnected, a trigger point in one area can cause, or "refer," pain in other areas as well. In fact, more than half of the time, pain related to trigger points will be felt in a place on the body that is separate from the trigger point. This pain (and the accompanying sensations like tingling and numbness) tends to occur in particular patterns, depending on which muscles have developed trigger points. Additionally, these patterns of pain often cover more than one region supplied by a spinal nerve.

It can be hard to know if the issue is coming from the spine or the muscle, which is why it's so important to treat both. This book will show you how, with methods to treat the spine *and* the muscle in question.

A Note on Medication

Some people with chronic pain use medication as part of their treatment plan. But with the realities of the opioid epidemic, many people are beginning to realize that it's important to consider other approaches for treating pain. You have such an approach in your hands. Perform these techniques as needed for non-opioid relief.

What Is Trigger Point Therapy?

Modern trigger point therapy owes its existence in large part to serendipity. Trigger point therapy pioneer Dr. Janet G. Travell leaned against a wall, and a coat hook poked the back of her shoulder. She noticed that it re-created the pain pattern she'd been experiencing in the front of her shoulder. She became determined to explain what she had experienced as well as how to treat it. She began to study the literature about pain, and what she discovered has helped people all over the world—including, now, you! Trigger point therapy is used as part of various disciplines, including massage, chiropractic, physical therapy, and even conventional medicine. Most importantly, people just like you have learned to use it to help themselves at home.

How Does Trigger Point Therapy Work?

Your nervous system loves when you apply pressure—*if* you do it properly. The right kind of pressure lengthens the shortened muscle fibers and causes the brain to release natural painkillers. Doing this consistently and keeping the area flexible makes the relief long-lasting. Adding in breathing techniques and movement principles can help keep the pain at bay.

The nerves in the skin over the painful region also respond positively to pressure (if it's held long enough). If the pressure is gentle, the brain learns that the region is receiving a pleasant touch and decides to lower the tension in the region. More intense pressure tends to make the brain release endorphins—your natural painkiller. That causes a significant decrease in pain as well. The brain loves pressure and stretch, and that's exactly what you'll be doing with the techniques you'll learn in this book. Happy brain, decreased pain. It's that simple.

Of course, re-irritating the region or re-creating the circumstances that caused the irritation in the first place can bring it back—but in this book, you'll learn what to do if that happens.

"It's All in Your Head"?

If you've ever had a serious injury or illness, you may have noticed that people can be very understanding about pain for a week or so. But if you're experiencing chronic pain, people begin to wonder if it's real or if it's "all in your head." In fact, they often say so out loud. These comments may even cause you to doubt your own experience. And going to the doctor often doesn't silence the critics, because a doctor who isn't looking for trigger points might tell you everything looks normal and they can't figure out what's wrong.

But just because people don't understand your pain doesn't mean it isn't real. Trigger points may be hard to detect with imaging tests or blood work, but they are the product of specific, concrete problems with muscles and nerves that have been mapped by physicians.

That said, there is always a mental component to pain. Every person with a nervous system sends constant information to their brain to allow it to decide what to do. The brain's output is determined not only by input from your body but also by emotions, past experiences, expectations, and your current understanding of what's wrong. Pain is not pain until the brain says it is. Physical trauma generally fires enough "danger signals" to your brain that it will tell you you're in pain. But you can—and with this book, will—use this understanding to give yourself effective treatment.

Does Trigger Point Therapy Hurt?

You're in control of how trigger point therapy feels. A trigger point is tender to the touch, but you get to determine the amount of pressure you apply. Generally speaking, the amount of discomfort you feel while working on your trigger points should be bearable, even comfortable. I've heard people describe the pain as "delicious."

If you like a higher level of pressure, you can press a bit more—just make sure it's not causing you to tighten up or hold your breath. If you have to fight the tightening of your muscles as they try to defend themselves from your touch, or if you're breathing like you're in childbirth, you might be overdoing it. Use your judgment within these guidelines.

Do I Need Professional Help?

Don't we all? But seriously—this book is all about you taking care of you. If you have chronic pain, self-care is likely a prominent part of your life. You are often your own best therapist, because only you know when you're on exactly the right place.

That said, professional help is wonderful, especially if your practitioner has both training and experience. If you can find help that works for you, by all means, use it.

The types of practitioners I recommend, in order:

Myofascial trigger point therapists are the best-trained professionals in this area. Trigger points are what they do. This is simply the best choice, bar none.

Neuromuscular massage therapists are trained to incorporate the treatment of trigger points in the context of a massage.

Chiropractors trained in Nimmo/receptor-tonus technique treat trigger points as an adjunct to their adjustments. They are often trained on this as students.

Physical therapists generally learn about trigger points as well as many other techniques. It's generally not their specialty, but some have availed themselves of trigger-point–specific training in addition to their primary education.

Beyond Massage

There are a few other effective methods of treating trigger points, but they can't be self-administered; they require a professional. Here are a few of these approaches to consider:

Spray and stretch involves spraying the muscle with a topical anesthetic while gently stretching it out. It feels amazing, yields impressive results, and was initially considered the workhorse of trigger point therapy. I especially love using this technique for migraines.

Dry needling looks like acupuncture and uses the same needles, but instead of being used on the acupuncture points of traditional Chinese medicine, the needles are used on trigger points. This is usually done by physical therapists.

Wet needling (trigger point injections) requires a physician to inject anesthetics into trigger points. There are a number of theories underlying how to use the needle. I have found this technique to be useful when the proper points have been chosen.

Frequency-specific microcurrent (FSM) involves treating various tissues with an electrical current that is not felt but that can have a profound effect on trigger points. Many different disciplines incorporate FSM.

Avazzia uses a probe to apply an electrical current to the skin over the trigger point. It often appears to decrease the sensitivity of the spot as well as restore the flexibility of the involved muscle. This is primarily used by massage therapists, chiropractors, acupuncturists, and physical therapists.

What to Expect

What can you expect from the methods in this book? Relief! Of course, there is no magic spell or silver bullet that can make your pain instantly disappear forever, but with regular treatment, you can expect to control, or at least decrease, your pain.

Keep in mind that you have to do the work in order to see what self-treatment can do for you and your pain. Relief may be short-lived if you have well-established trigger points or other conditions that keep irritating your muscles and nerves. Continued daily work may be needed, but it's worth the effort—if a given massage technique got rid of your pain for 30 minutes this time, it may work for 60 minutes next time.

People who practice self-treatment often experience a significant decrease in their pain, which improves their ability to function from day to day. Many people do this with little, if any, need for medication or professional treatment. It's a huge blessing to those who have been trapped in their own body by horrible, unrelenting pain. People love the independence that self-management of trigger points provides.

CHAPTER TWO

Essential Pain Relief Techniques

The previous chapter gave you essential information about what trigger points are and how they work. This chapter will give you the basic tools you need to perform trigger point therapy on yourself at home. It will go over proper massage techniques, what equipment to use, and even mental approaches you can take. Then, in part 2, you'll learn how to apply these techniques and tools to help bring you relief from pain.

Massage Techniques

If you've been experiencing acute or chronic myofascial pain, you've probably tried massaging yourself or getting a professional massage. You may have been disappointed to find that you didn't see a big difference in pain. That's because there's more to treating trigger points than just rubbing at a sore spot and hoping for the best. There are certain techniques that provide the best results. For most trigger points, I start treatment with paraspinal massage and nerve flossing, move on to applying compression massage to the trigger point, and finish with gentle motions known as "Swedish movements." Let's take a closer look at all these techniques.

Paraspinal Massage

To put it in simple terms, your nerves carry information about sensations (pressure, temperature, and so on) between your brain and the rest of your body by traveling through your spine. Your spine consists of 33 vertebrae divided into five regions: cervical (in the neck), thoracic (in the upper back), lumbar (in the lower back), sacral (in the hips/pelvis), and coccyx (the tailbone). Each region connects different parts of your body back to your brain.

Because of the way these spinal regions communicate with different areas of your body, massaging specific muscles alongside your spine—known as the paraspinal muscles—can help treat pain in other areas of your body. For example, the nerves that supply your trapezius muscles run through the fifth, sixth, and seventh vertebrae in the cervical region ("C5" through "C7,"

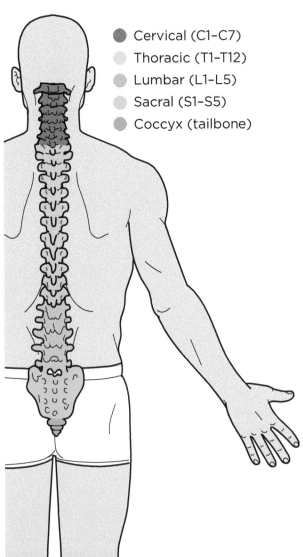

● Cervical (C1–C7)
○ Thoracic (T1–T12)
○ Lumbar (L1–L5)
○ Sacral (S1–S5)
● Coccyx (tailbone)

for short). So if you have pain in your trapezius, massaging the paraspinal muscles next to those vertebrae in your lower neck is an important part of treatment. In fact, it's usually the first step in treating any muscle pain. Part 2 of this book will include instructions on how to figure out which paraspinals to massage in order to treat the area where you're experiencing pain.

Nerve Flossing

Nerve flossing, also known as "nerve gliding" or "neural gliding," is an amazing practice developed in physical therapy that is actually considered a form of friction massage. Nerves are essentially thin cables of nerve fibers, and they have a range of motion, just like muscles. If you perform certain movements (for example, flexing and extending your wrist), the nerves slide back and forth, just like a piece of floss would slide back and forth between teeth. (Except you don't need to buy the floss!)

This helps loosen up the nerve, giving it a better range of motion and reducing pain. I find that if I floss a nerve before treating a nearby trigger point, the muscle is more relaxed and responds better and longer to treatment. I often have my clients nerve floss in my office prior to treatment as well as at home between treatments.

Nerve flossing looks different depending on which nerve you're targeting, but it usually involves a gentle, non-painful, back-and-forth movement of some body part. Different nerve flossing techniques, useful for different trigger point areas, will be covered throughout part 2 of this book.

Finding the Trigger Point

Before you can massage a trigger point, you have to be able to find it. Here's the best technique for locating a trigger point:

1. Most trigger points can be located by slightly stretching the muscle causing the pain. The pictures of the pain patterns in each chapter of this book will help you know which muscle to test for tightness. The spot where you feel a pull or tightness while doing a simple stretch is usually the location of the trigger point. Most entries in part 2 of this book include a stretch test to help you find the area where the trigger point is located.

2. Locate the tender muscle band by using your fingers to probe across the muscle where you felt the pull of the stretch. I like to think of probing the muscle fibers as running my fingers over a keyboard. If I feel a guitar string, that's the tender band. These bands can be narrow or wide. This part of the technique may take some practice, but it's really helpful.

3. Once you have located the tender muscle band, sink your fingers gently into the muscle and rub your fingers across its fibers, searching for a tender spot. It can be anywhere from the size of a BB to the size of a bean. That's your target—press there!

Note: Some muscles, including the sternocleidomastoid, brachioradialis, and hamstrings, need to be squeezed in addition to or instead of being pressed. You can rub the muscle between your thumb and fingers to find the tender spot.

Trigger Point Compression Massage

Once you've located the trigger point, apply direct pressure to that point and hold it for 10 to 60 seconds—whatever feels best for you. If that sounds simple, that's because it is! You can just use your fingers, but most of the time I recommend using a variety of self-massage tools instead (see page 18). The muscles in your hands are delicate, and if you're practicing self-massage on a regular basis, they can get worn out surprisingly quickly.

Remember that the pressure can be gentle or firm. I've heard many people say that they like the sensation somewhere between "pleasure" and "pain." The pleasure comes from knowing you're on the right spot and feeling the muscle fibers softening as pressure is applied. The trick is to not change your breathing or tighten the muscle once you begin applying pressure.

Self-treatment quickly becomes an art form in which you are both canvas and painter. You get to know your own body and just what it needs. Pain is just your body asking you for attention.

Remember that a trigger point in one muscle can refer pain to an entirely different muscle. This means that much of the time, you'll have to massage somewhere other than where you're feeling the pain. The entries in part 2 of this book will help you find the spots where you should apply pressure, even when they're not the places you might expect.

Swedish Movements

You may have heard of or even experienced Swedish massage. Originally called "the Swedish movement cure," it involved doing a few simple range-of-motion movements with the affected area in addition to the massage treatment. It thrived in the United States between 1850 and 1920, but when the polio epidemic hit, people began to focus more on strengthening exercises, and the simple movement aspect was largely lost.

But not completely lost! I consider post-massage Swedish movements an essential part of pain treatment. Whereas the physical therapy you might be familiar with focuses on strengthening and, to an extent, stretching, Swedish movements were developed to improve circulation. They are used here as a gentle, painless way to focus on retraining the nervous system in the range of motion that's available for a given muscle.

Let's go over the basic breakdown of a Swedish movement, followed by a more in-depth explanation of how each movement works.

The basic breakdown:

1. Start in a neutral position.

2. Move the muscle in question from the neutral position toward a fully lengthened position. You don't want to hold any of these movements for a prolonged period of time. Keep moving—this is not a traditional stretch!

3. Return to neutral and pause briefly, for about one second.

4. After the pause, fully shorten the muscle in question—but this time, don't hold it.

5. Return to neutral. Pause for one second again.

6. Repeat four more times for a total of five repetitions.

Now let's go over a specific example. Let's say you have pain in your latissimus dorsi, the muscles in your back commonly called the "lats." The associated Swedish movement would look like this:

1. Start in a neutral position, sitting or standing with your arms hanging at your sides, your palms open, and your thumbs pointing forward.

2. Take the arm on the treatment side (the side where you're feeling pain), and bring it straight out in front of you, slowly tracing an arc

toward the ceiling until your arm is over your shoulder and pointing behind you. This is the fully lengthened position.

3. Slowly retracing the same path with your arm, return to the neutral position. Pause.

4. Now move your arm slowly in the opposite direction until it's extended behind you. (You won't have as much range of motion in this direction.) This is the fully shortened position.

5. Return to neutral. Pause.

6. Repeat four more times for a total of five repetitions.

That's it! It may seem simple, or not as "serious" as getting a massage, but don't skip it. This is an essential part of the treatment. It helps the benefits of trigger point therapy take effect and last over time.

The early Swedish movement authors recommended four to six repetitions of the movements as part of the massage treatment. Dr. Janet Travell emphasized the importance of doing at least three range-of-motion movements to retrain the muscle. Dr. Gabriel Sella, an authority on biofeedback, recommends five repetitions to retrain movements, based on his database of nearly 6,000 tests. I like five.

The Right Tools for the Job

Any carpenter or mechanic will tell you that the most important part of their work is getting the right tool for the job. Here are some tools that you should consider investing in, depending on your particular issue. My favorite tool is whichever one I need for my current problem.

Your Hands

Most of us keep two hands with us at all times. They are often the first tool you take out of your treatment bag. There are a number of things to keep in mind when using your hands to self-treat trigger points.

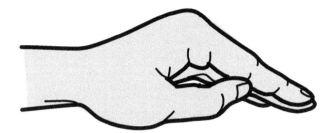

- Keep your nails trimmed.

- Never press hard with your fingers—you have other tools for that. Press lightly; your body can learn to love gentle pressure.

- Keep your wrist straight and your fingers slightly curved when you apply pressure, like in the image above. Your fingers will thank you.

- At the end of your wrist, on the same side as your pinky finger, is a bony little knob. It's called the pisiform bone, and it fits like a lock in a key for some muscles. If you're treating a muscle where it feels like the pisiform bone might work, give it a try—it's a real thumb saver.

- If at all possible, don't use your thumbs. They're hard to help once you've abused them, and hard pressure is abuse.

- It's not all about your fingers; above your hand is an elbow, which can be great for applying pressure. In part 2, I'll tell you when to use it.

- Use leverage whenever possible. It saves you.

Hooks and Knobs

Hooks and knobs are simply amazing for self-massage. They save your hands and can get to regions that you just can't reach or put enough pressure on by yourself. There are many to choose from. Here are a few of my favorites.

THE BIG BEND BACKNOBBER
To get in the region just beside your spine where those tiny little para-spinal muscles reside, you can't beat the Big Bend Backnobber, an elegant

S-shaped tool from The Pressure Positive Company. The large end fits around your body and the hook uses the ground (or your favorite chair) as a fulcrum to get the short paraspinal muscles. As you'll see in part 2, I recommend treating those muscles as a first step before treating your problem muscles. That makes this tool really important.

THE THUMBBY AND THE KNOBBLE

The Thumbby and the Knobble are small knobs that you can use to apply more pressure without abusing your fingers. The Thumbby is made of rubber and can stick to a wall so that you can lean against it. It looks nothing like a thumb, but it feels like one when you use it to self-massage. Both tools feel great in your palm.

THE ACUMASSEUR

An amazing variant on the knob is the Acumasseur. It looks kind of like a giant nutcracker with golf balls at the top. It's great to trap a muscle knot between the balls and squeeze for blessed relief.

Balls

Balls were my first tool. A ball can be placed on the floor or behind you on a hard chair; you can also drop them in tube socks or pantyhose to keep them from rolling away. (I know a therapist who put tennis balls in purple pantyhose and sold them as "purple pain erasers.") Find a tender nodule, place it against the ball, and ease your weight into it. Avoid pressing so hard that you tighten the muscles or have to breathe through the pain.

Most people start with tennis balls. A racquetball is great for higher up on the back. A ball that is larger than a grapefruit but smaller than a soccer ball allows gentle treatment to the deeper muscles of the belly and can be found for cheap in almost any toy store.

Another ball-based tool is the Original Worm, which is essentially four balls held together in a soft neoprene case with no rough edges. You can hold it or place it wherever you need to. Just lean into it.

Rollers

I usually prefer holding pressure on a trigger point, but if you're one of those people who enjoys rolling out your pain, then a portable roller called the Tiger Tail was made for you. It feels amazing to roll it over your legs on every side. They have larger rollers for your back, too. I recommend rolling very slowly for the full effect.

Pain Relief Gel

Another amazing tool is a gel from DERM Creations called O_2 Derm Relief. It's a method of getting oxygen into your skin and the tissues beneath. I put it on the spinal nerve supply and on the trigger point. The muscle in question relaxes in seconds and becomes more responsive to treatment. I don't work or travel without it.

Safety First

There are a few safety tips to keep in mind when practicing trigger point therapy at home.

Don't massage a pulse. Be careful when massaging the front of your neck (where your carotid artery is located), your groin (where your femoral artery is located), or anywhere else you feel a pulse. Massaging a pulse has the potential to interrupt your blood flow or loosen any plaque in your arteries, potentially leading to a heart attack or stroke.

Don't massage your lymph nodes. Those are the small, bean-sized nodes located in your neck, armpits, groin, and elsewhere. Don't mistake them for muscle knots or trigger points, which are much smaller. And if they're swollen, have your doctor check them out.

Don't massage any red or swollen areas. You'll likely just make the inflammation worse. This is especially important if the affected area is in the calf. If you're experiencing any of these symptoms, see your doctor.

Watch out for "lightning" pain or throbbing. Trigger point pain is usually deep, dull, and aching. If you have more acute pain, take it to your doctor. There may well be trigger points involved, but the primary cause is usually something else, and someone who goes by "doctor" should probably be involved in your treatment.

Other Approaches to Pain Relief

We've talked about the basics of treating trigger points with physical approaches like nerve flossing, compression massage, and various massage tools. As important as that all is, there's much more to the picture. We experience pain through the nervous system, so to control pain, it's especially important to calm the nervous system. There are a number of both physical and mental techniques you can use—here are some of my favorites.

Breathing Exercises

You've probably noticed that breathing deeply can help you calm down, but did you know it actually changes the chemistry in your body? If you're breathing too shallowly due to anxiety, stress, or bad breathing habits, or if you're just not breathing enough, then your body is not converting enough of the oxygen you inhale to CO_2, which can raise the pH of your blood from 7.4 to 7.5 or 7.6. This is called hypocapnia, and it has a vasoconstrictive effect, meaning it narrows your blood vessels and restricts normal blood flow. As a consequence, your muscles and fasciae can spasm, twitch, feel weak, and hurt. So breathing exercises aren't just a good way to relax—they very literally get your blood flowing and help prevent and treat trigger points.

My favorite breathing exercise is simple but effective:

- Inhale through your nose for a count of six.

- Hold for a count of one.

- Slowly exhale for a count of four.

- Continue for three minutes.

Here's another simple but effective breathing exercise that I find especially useful for going to sleep:

- Visualize a whiteboard.

- Inhale as you envision yourself writing the number 0.

- Slowly and completely exhale as you envision yourself erasing the number 0.

- Repeat with the numbers 1 through 9.

Fidget, Wiggle, and Squirm

When part of our body isn't getting enough oxygen because of a lack of blood flow, we instinctively move to allow blood to flow back into the area. This stops the discomfort until we naturally need to move again.

The problem arises when we inhibit this instinctive movement because we think others might be watching and could criticize us or think we're weird. So we sit still and allow the discomfort to increase. We really need to get over this! Fidget as much as you need to fidget to feel comfortable.

Slapping

When you have chronic pain, the brain tends to become either hyper-irritable or accustomed to ramped-up neurological input. This is called "accommodation." In short, the brain stops paying attention. The soft tissues in your body tighten up, receiving less blood flow. Less blood flow means less oxygen reaches the skin, nerves, and muscles in the tightened area. And in the absence of oxygen, we often have pain.

Gentle, painless slapping all over your body brings the brain's attention to the areas it's trying to ignore. It also increases blood flow for a period of time, which gives us the ability to move more freely and painlessly. It requires no equipment and can be done almost anywhere. You can even see some martial artists and Olympic athletes doing it. There's not much scientific research on this technique, but I've yet to see it fail.

If you feel like spending money, you can also buy a special brush for "dry brushing" the skin. It works the same way. (I get the same results toweling off after a shower—but I can't exactly do that at work!)

Self-care is absolutely essential if you want to get better. Just lying on a treatment table and getting "fixed" rarely works. You need to pay attention to your overall health to create an environment for your nervous system and muscles to downregulate. Getting enough sleep, eating a balanced diet, and taking some time to relax aren't just things to cross off your to-do list—they're effective pain-management techniques.

Understanding What's Happening

A huge part of dealing with pain is understanding what's happening inside your body. Too often, people worry that their pain is caused by something unknown. They think something scary is lurking in their tissues. They expect the worst and let those thoughts cycle through their brain. This is harmful, and it needs to stop.

If you've been through the differential diagnosis process by seeing many doctors and have had a litany of scans and tests, it's highly unlikely that there is some hidden process responsible for your pain. Scar tissue forms within two to three months after an injury (although it takes about a year to fully mature). If the cause of your pain is something that can be picked up by X-rays, CT scans, or MRIs, then you'll see it in the results. But the truth is that the majority of people scanned with these technologies don't find any issues related to their pain. It's most likely that you have a sensitive nervous system, irritated nerves, and/or trigger points—not that you're at the mercy of a mysterious disease that you'll never figure out how to treat.

Additionally, there are just a few types of soft tissue in your body. They all have medical names in Latin and Greek that can make them sound scarier than they need to be. I think diagnosis needs to be demystified. Doctors should name a body part, say it hurts, and maybe why it hurts. It doesn't need to be intimidating. Just understanding what's going on with your pain and knowing that you have the tools to help is huge. This book is chock-full of ideas and directions to help you deal with your pain. You have some pretty substantial control.

Retraining Your Brain

Now that you know that your pain issues are likely related to irritated nerves and muscles, you can stop focusing on the unknown and start thinking about your pain in a way that doesn't stress you out and make the problem even worse. Some techniques that can help:

- Your doctor or therapist may have told you what muscles are causing the biggest issues for you. Look them up in this book and learn about them. Where do they send pain?

- If you find a treatment or technique that helps, then you know to do it again. Keep doing the same thing that got results.

- I've known people to copy their pain pattern or print it out off the internet and put it up where they can see it. It reminds them of what the issue is and stops them from catastrophizing and jumping to conclusions about the worst-case scenario.

- Moving the region where pain is normally experienced through a smaller, pain-free motion (and repeating this often) can help change the signals between your nerves and your brain. It causes your brain to realize that movement is safe.

- Visualizing yourself doing activities in a pain-free manner can help retrain your brain so that it does not continue to output the same reaction to circumstances.

Helpful Habits

Developing habits that keep our minds calm and our muscles and nerves relaxed helps keep our pain at bay. Here are some of my favorites:

- Set a kitchen timer and put it on the other side of the room. Set it so you have to get up every 20 minutes to reset it. This keeps you from sitting still for too long, which is helpful for your muscles.

- Make sure the chair you sit in fits you. Ideally, your feet can rest on the floor, your back will be supported, and your elbows will reach the armrests.

- Go to sleep and wake up at the same time every day.

- Make sure to communicate clearly, often, and intimately with those you love.

- An active social life is very important. Places of worship, clubs, and civic organizations get you out in public and into relationships. This has a huge impact on pain.

- Find a sport or movement discipline that interests you. I like martial arts and ballroom dance. It keeps your muscles working and can be fun.

- The breathing exercises on page 22 do wonders to downregulate your nervous system.

- By calming your nerves, the nerve flossing techniques throughout part 2 often calm your brain, too.

- When pressing on trigger points, it is often calming to just barely touch the areas and hold for two to four minutes. The brain actually learns from lighter touch over a long period of time.

Tips and Tricks

Here are a few tips I've discovered over the years to help make your trigger point therapy more effective:

- When pain is really irritating, people tend to forget the important details that are often the most helpful. The cure: a list! Create a one-page bulleted list of what you need to do to treat your trigger points. Keep copies in a few important places where you can get your hands on them quickly. I've used the refrigerator, a wall next to my desk, and my phone. You can also create a list on your smartphone. Your solutions may vary, but make that list.

- Along the same lines, you may want to photocopy or bookmark the pages you use most in this book so you can access them easily. You could also take pictures of the relevant pages and store them in an easy-to-access folder on your phone.

- It's easy to overtreat yourself when you're in a hurry or in a lot of pain. But that can lead to more pain. Treat one to two times a day per region—no more. Remember to breathe and move. Use heat or a hot bath. (If a particular muscle is really irritable, an ice pack or bag of frozen peas can calm it down, but I suggest starting with heat.)

- Self-treatment is important, but timing and frequency are highly individual. Some people need to treat their trigger points daily just to get by. Others find success doing it only a few times a week. It's wise to treat your trigger points often enough to see that you're making and maintaining progress, but don't get stuck on the idea that you need to meet an arbitrary goal.

- Don't get so involved in physical activities—like mopping a floor or hammering a nail—that you push yourself into pain. Stop and take care of you. This helps to ensure that you don't pay for it later. And just because you don't have time for a full treatment doesn't mean you can't do something quick for relief if you're feeling pain. Do what you can. Your body will thank you for it.

- Focusing on something you enjoy often distracts your brain from the pain, and distraction is a potent pain reliever. Try to find an activity you love that you can do regularly, like volunteering with a local charity.

- You can usually tone down the pain considerably by doing the breathing exercises on page 22.

- Pain increases when you're stressed. It can be really important to avoid those stressors when possible. Because of this, you may find it important to avoid the news or social media at times.

- Sleep is incredibly important, so if you struggle with insomnia or sleep quality, it's important to look for solutions. Engaging in basic sleep hygiene really improves the quality of sleep. Keep your bedroom a place you use exclusively for sleep or adult activity—not discussing finances, hanging out with your kids, or watching TV.

PART TWO

What to Do

YOU'VE ARRIVED! NOW YOU GET TO APPLY THE information you learned in part 1. (Don't cheat—make sure you read part 1 first!)

Here's how to use part 2:

First, consult the Symptom Index on page 186 or flip to the chapter that pertains to your pain—for example, if you have pain in your head or face, go to the chapter on the head and face—and find the appropriate entry.

The entry for each muscle (or muscle group) will give you the information you need to treat that area, starting with an image that shows you the approximate spot where the trigger points would be located as well as the associated pain pattern. Note that the trigger points highlighted on the image aren't meant to indicate exact areas; trigger points are very small and can be located anywhere within the muscle. Also note that although an illustration may only show trigger points on one side of the body, they can show up on either side or on both sides at the same time. I'll refer to the side experiencing the pain as the "treatment side" and the side not experiencing pain as the "non-treatment side."

Next, the entry will tell you where you'll feel pain if you have trigger points in a given muscle, as well as other symptoms you might be experiencing due to those trigger points. It will also list common reasons why those trigger points develop.

Most importantly, it'll walk you through four important treatment steps for each muscle.

Step 1: Treat the Spine

The nerves that run through your body connect back to your brain through your spine. If you massage next to the correct part of the spine, you can treat the pain in all the muscles that connect there. Step 1 will tell you which vertebrae the muscle's nerve supply runs through so you can massage the paraspinal muscles (the muscles directly adjacent to the spine) in the correct place.

Step 2: Floss the Nerve

"Flossing" a nerve (sliding it back and forth, kind of like a piece of floss) reduces irritation in the nerve and thus reduces pain in the muscles it supplies. Step 2 will tell you what motion to use to floss the nerve that supplies the muscle in question.

Step 3: Treat the Trigger Points

Step 3 will walk you through how to locate tender spots and apply pressure with gentle compression massage.

Step 4: Gently Move

Remember the Swedish movements from chapter 2? They improve circulation and help retrain your brain to understand that the muscle in question still has a range of motion, even if it's in pain. This step will show you which movements to utilize.

Each entry will also include a list of other muscles to treat. Remember, trigger points in one area can refer pain to a completely different area, so sometimes you'll have to treat a muscle in a place you might not have expected. This list will let you know where to start.

Let's do it!

CHAPTER THREE

Head and Face

Do you struggle with pain in your head, face, or jaw? It's very common for the pain associated with headaches and temporomandibular joint (TMJ) dysfunction to come from trigger points—although the relevant trigger points often aren't in the head and face but rather in the sternocleido-mastoid muscles in the neck or the trapezius muscles in the shoulders. This chapter will instruct you on where and how to massage to get relief from pain in your head and face.

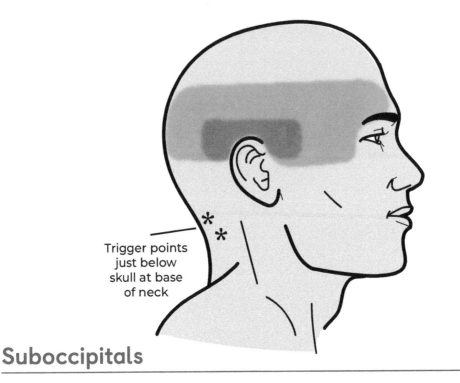

Trigger points just below skull at base of neck

Suboccipitals

Where it hurts: This pain goes right through your entire head and often seems to settle tight behind the eye.

You might also be experiencing: Full-body tightness.

It's often caused by: Whiplash injuries, chronic stress.

Step 1: **Treat the Spine**

• Using your fingers, apply pressure to the deep paraspinal muscles in the gutter just beside the C1 vertebra at the very top of the neck. Don't press on the bone itself.

• Apply pressure to both sides of the spine for 10 to 90 seconds.

Step 2: **Floss the Nerve**

• Do the Slumping for Health nerve floss (page 132) to floss the suboccipital nerve.

Step 3: **Treat the Trigger Points**

• Lie on your back, tuck your chin toward your chest, and gently probe for tender spots in the center of the area where your skull meets your spine.

• Apply gentle pressure to each tender spot for 10 to 90 seconds.

Step 4: **Gently Move**

- Start by sitting or standing in a neutral position.

- Lengthen the muscles by gently tucking your chin toward your chest. Return to neutral.

- Shorten the muscles by gently jutting your head forward. Return to neutral.

- Repeat a total of five times.

Other muscles to treat: The trapezius (page 56), the sternocleidomastoid (page 50), and occasionally the pectorals (pages 114 and 116) can refer pain to the suboccipitals.

Safety First

If I could treat only one part of the body, it would be the suboccipitals. The entire body usually relaxes after treating it. However, this region needs to be treated *very* carefully, if at all. Here's how to determine whether it's safe to treat your suboccipitals yourself or if you need to consult a doctor:

- Lean forward and put your elbows on your knees.

- Put your head in your hands and open your eyes.

- Have someone look and see if your eyes begin to "bounce," moving rapidly from side to side or up and down while you're looking in a single direction. If they do, it can be a sign of a serious health issue, so it's time to get to your doctor's office. Do not self-treat.

- If your eyes don't begin to bounce, press gently on the suboccipitals. If you feel like you're blacking out or if you feel strange sensations like numbness, tingling, or weakness going down your arm, do not self-treat. Go see your doctor.

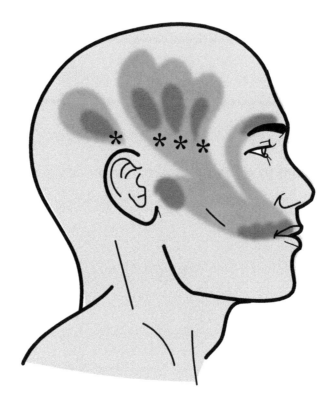

Temporalis

Where it hurts: The temple and the part of the jaw below the temple.

You might also be experiencing: Pain or sensitivity in your teeth. A police officer who had developed trigger points on his temporalis after being rear-ended thought I had fixed his toothache after I treated this muscle!

It's often caused by: Trigger points in your trapezius and/or sternocleido-mastoid muscles. Sometimes it's irritated by dental issues or a blow to the head.

Step 1: Treat the Spine

- Because this muscle is supplied by a nerve in the head, it does not require a paraspinal treatment.

Step 2: Floss the Nerve

- Use the Jig Jaw nerve floss (page 46) to floss the trigeminal nerve.

Step 3: Treat the Trigger Points

- Open your mouth wide and feel the muscles on the outside to sense where the tightness is. That's the spot you want to target.

- Press gently in a line about a finger's width above the bone between the outside edge of your eye and your ear, looking for tender spots.

- Apply pressure to any tender spots, holding each one for between 10 and 90 seconds.

Step 4: Gently Move

- Gently yawn a total of five times.

Other muscles to treat: The trapezius (page 56), sternocleidomastoid (page 50), and masseter (page 38).

Tip: Gentleness is the key when treating this muscle. Pressing too hard can cause a headache.

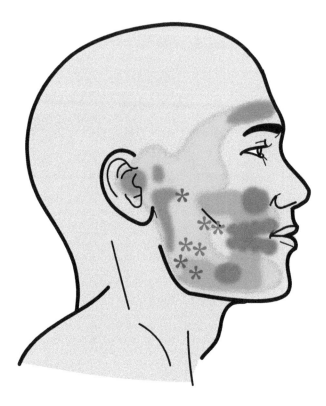

Masseter

Where it hurts: In the jaw, and often in the forehead and sinus region.

You might also be experiencing: A feeling of tightness when opening your mouth wide, ringing in your ears.

It's often caused by: Trigger points in your trapezius and/or sternocleido-mastoid, dental issues, or a blow to the head.

Step 1: **Treat the Spine**

- Because this muscle is supplied by a nerve in the head, it does not require a paraspinal treatment.

Step 2: **Floss the Nerve**

- Use the Jig Jaw nerve floss (page 46) to floss the trigeminal nerve.

Step 3: **Treat the Trigger Points**

- Open your jaw and feel where it's tight. Probe this short muscle gently, looking for tender spots.

- Apply and hold pressure on each tender spot for 10 to 90 seconds.

Step 4: **Gently Move**

- Gently yawn a total of five times.

Other muscles to treat: The trapezius (page 56), sternocleidomastoid (page 50), and temporalis (page 36).

Tip: Cracking ice or opening nuts with your teeth may irritate this muscle—so don't do it. When I had masseter pain after a car crash, it made chewing gum or eating tough, chewy foods very painful. I'd recommend not doing either until after you've treated the muscle and recovered.

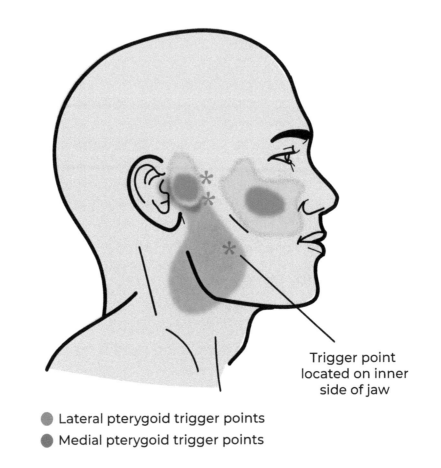

Trigger point located on inner side of jaw

● Lateral pterygoid trigger points
● Medial pterygoid trigger points

Medial and Lateral Pterygoids

Where it hurts: The jaw and sinus regions. If you thought it was sinus pressure but cold medicine didn't help, trigger points in this area are quite possibly the culprit.

You might also be experiencing: Trouble moving your jaw from side to side, a visible zigzag movement of your jaw you can see in the mirror, or popping and clicking in your jaw. One patient related with tears how, after treatment, her family members no longer made fun of the sounds her jaw made when she ate.

It's often caused by: Trigger points in your trapezius and/or sternocleido-mastoid, dental issues, or a blow to the head.

Step 1: Treat the Spine

- Because this muscle is supplied by a nerve in the head, it does not require a paraspinal treatment.

Step 2: Floss the Nerve

- Use the Jig Jaw nerve floss (page 46) to floss the trigeminal nerve.

Step 3: Treat the Trigger Points

- Roll your finger under the end of the bone at the back of the jaw, looking for tender spots on the inside of your jaw. You can also feel in front of the jaw joint (TMJ) when it is open. Press in and forward, then in and downward. (This is all done externally—don't look for tender spots inside the mouth.)

- Hold the pressure on any tender spots for 10 to 90 seconds.

Step 4: Gently Move

- Gently yawn a total of five times.

Other muscles to treat: The trapezius (page 56), sternocleidomastoid (page 50), masseter (page 38), and temporalis (page 36).

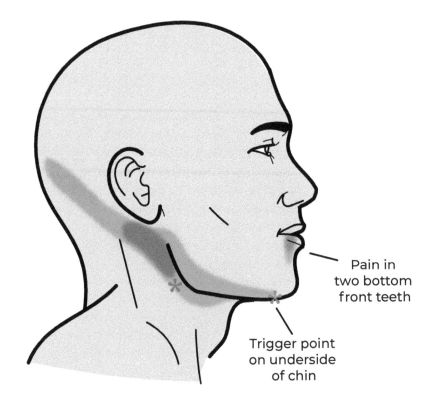

Pain in
two bottom
front teeth

Trigger point
on underside
of chin

Digastric

Where it hurts: Your bottom two front teeth as well as below the back of your jaw and ear.

You might also be experiencing: Ear pain.

It's often caused by: Whiplash injuries and grinding your teeth.

Step 1: **Treat the Spine**

- Because this muscle is supplied by nerves in the head, it does not require a paraspinal treatment.

Step 2: **Floss the Nerve**

- Use the Jig Jaw nerve floss (page 46) to floss the facial and trigeminal nerves.

Step 3: **Treat the Trigger Points**

- Feel around under your jaw in the front for tender spots.

- Apply and hold pressure to each tender spot for 10 to 90 seconds.

Step 4: **Gently Move**

- Sit or stand in a neutral position.

- Lengthen the muscle by gently tilting your head back and looking up toward the ceiling. Don't crane your neck or tilt your head all the way back—just look upward. Return to neutral.

- Shorten the muscle by tilting your head (not your neck) down to look at the floor. Return to neutral.

- Repeat a total of five times.

Other muscles to treat: The sternocleidomastoid (page 50).

Tip: A night guard can be useful for people who grind their teeth.

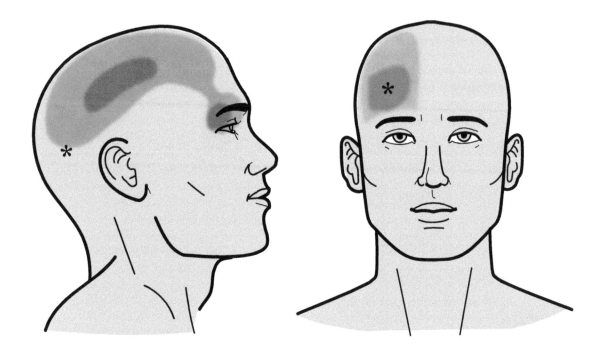

Occipitofrontalis

Where it hurts: The occipitalis (the back of the head), the frontalis (the forehead), and the scalp in between. This muscle is unusual in that it doesn't send pain to another part of the body—it only creates pain in the area where it's located.

You might also be experiencing: Pain in the back of your head while lying down on a pillow.

It's often caused by: Falling and hitting the head, or being hit in the head. Even wearing a helmet when sparring or riding a bike won't keep these muscles from developing trigger points.

Step 1: Treat the Spine

- Use your fingers to press the paraspinal muscles next to the first three vertebrae in your upper neck. Don't press on the bone itself.

- Apply pressure to any tender spots for 10 to 60 seconds each.

Step 2: Floss the Nerve

- Do the Jig Jaw nerve floss (page 46) to floss the facial nerve.

- After you have completed the last jaw movement, stick out your tongue and move it slowly from side to side, then raise and lower your eyebrows.

- Repeat the whole sequence a total of 10 times.

Step 3: Treat the Trigger Points

- Use your fingers to slowly and gently touch your forehead, your scalp, and the back of your head, searching for tender spots.

- When you find a tender spot, apply gentle pressure for 10 to 90 seconds.

Step 4: Gently Move

- This muscle does not have an associated movement.

Other muscles to treat: The sternocleidomastoid (page 50) and trapezius (page 56).

Tip: Be gentle! These muscles are very thin and do not require much pressure.

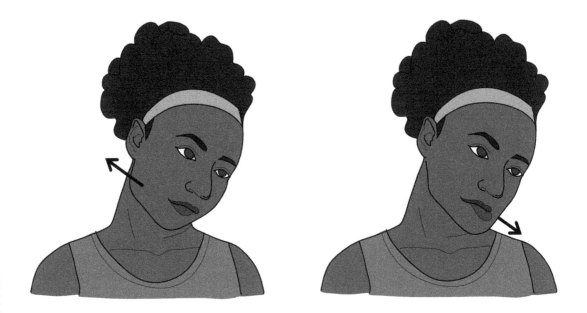

NERVE FLOSS: Jig Jaw

This movement flosses the trigeminal and facial nerves, which helps relieve pain in several muscles in the head and face, including the occipitofrontalis (page 44), temporalis (page 36), and pterygoids (page 40).

Instructions

- Start in a neutral standing or sitting position. Your head should be in a relaxed but upright position, looking forward.

- Tuck your chin in and bring your ear straight down toward your shoulder, away from the side being treated. Turn your head down, looking toward your opposite pants pocket. Slide your jaw slowly from side to side.

- This motion needs to be done slowly. Repeat 10 times.

CHAPTER FOUR

Neck and Shoulders

Trigger points in the neck and shoulders can refer pain to so many different areas. Two of the most important muscles related to headaches are located here, for example, and if you have pain and numbness going down your arms, then you might want to spend some quality time with this chapter. If you have a rotator cuff injury, you will want to treat trigger points related to the problem in addition to the injury itself. Traumas like car accidents, falls, and work-related injuries often lead people to develop trigger points in this area, though they can also have more mundane causes, like bad posture or sitting at a desk all day. Daily self-treatment can lead to long-lasting relief.

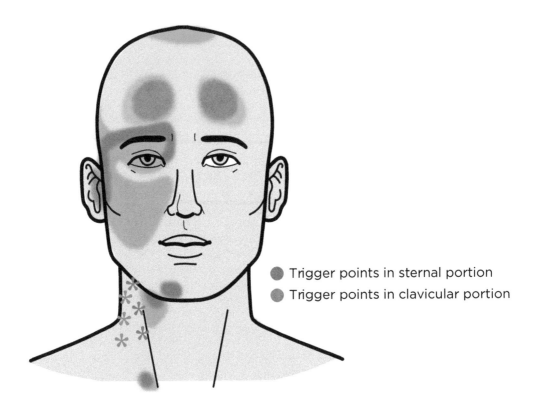

Trigger points in sternal portion
Trigger points in clavicular portion

Sternocleidomastoid

Where it hurts: The back and top of the head, around the eye, the top of the breastbone, the forehead, the ear, and behind the ear.

You might also be experiencing: Ringing in the ears, runny nose, dizziness, and narrowing of your eyelids.

It's often caused by: Prolonged stress, sticking your head forward.

Step 1: Treat the Spine

- Using your fingers, an Acumasseur, or a Thumbby, apply pressure to the paraspinal muscles alongside the first four vertebrae in the upper neck.

- Hold the pressure for 10 to 90 seconds on both sides of the spine.

Step 2: Floss the Nerve

- Perform the Shoulder Back, Head Forward nerve floss (page 74) to floss the spinal accessory nerve.

Step 3: Treat the Trigger Points

- Using the hand on the non-treatment side, reach across your body to lift and gently pinch the sternal portion of the muscle (the part that connects to your sternum, indicated by the trigger points in pink).

- Reach slightly farther across to do the same thing for the clavicular portion of the muscle (the part that connects to your clavicle, or collarbone, indicated by the trigger points in orange). (Sometimes this portion is slippery. I use a tissue to hold it.)

- Hold the squeezes for 10 to 90 seconds per tender spot. Be gentle—it's easy to squeeze too hard and increase the pain.

Step 4: Gently Move

- Start in a neutral sitting or standing position.

- Lengthen the muscle by turning your head to the treatment side as far as is comfortably possible for you. Once your head is turned, drop your chin down and look behind you and up. Return to neutral.

- Shorten the muscle by repeating the same movement on the other side.

- Repeat the movement a total of five times.

Other muscles to treat: The pectoralis major (page 114), pectoralis minor (page 116), and trapezius (page 56). You might also try the psoas (page 140), rectus femoris (page 138), and tensor fasciae latae (page 136).

Tip: Be careful when massaging the front of your neck. Remember not to apply pressure directly on a pulse!

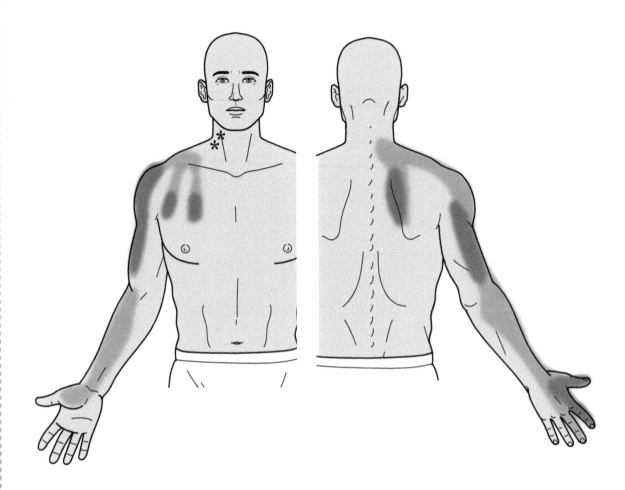

Scalenes

Where it hurts: Between the shoulder blades. You might also experience pain down the arm or, in really bad cases, in the chest.

You might also be experiencing: Waking with your hands swollen, numbness/tingling down the arms.

It's often caused by: A whiplash injury, sleeping on your side with a pillow that's too thick.

Step 1: Treat the Spine

- Using an Acumasseur, Thumbby, or similar tool, apply pressure to the paraspinal muscles right next to the C2–C7 vertebrae in your lower neck.

Step 2: **Floss the Nerve**

- Start in a neutral standing or sitting position with your head in a relaxed but upright position, looking forward.

- Tilt your head to the non-treatment side, bringing the ear toward the shoulder. Return to neutral.

- Now tilt your head the other way, bringing your ear toward the shoulder on the treatment side. Hold your arms so that your inner elbow is turned outward, and move to the opposite side. Return to neutral.

- Repeat a total of 10 times.

Step 3: **Treat the Trigger Points**

- Using the hand on the non-treatment side, reach across your body and gently grasp the sternocleidomastoid (see page 50) on the treatment side. Roll your fingers behind the outer edge and you'll be touching your scalene.

- Apply pressure on any tender spots for 10 to 90 seconds each. Remember to be careful when massaging the front of your neck— don't apply pressure directly on a pulse.

Step 4: **Gently Move**

- Start in a neutral seated or standing position.

- Lengthen the muscle by tilting your head to the side so that you're bringing the ear toward the non-treatment shoulder. Return to neutral.

- Shorten the muscle by tilting your head the other way, bringing your ear toward the shoulder on the treatment side. Return to neutral.

- Repeat a total of five times.

Other muscles to treat: The upper trapezius (page 56), pectoralis major (page 114), and pectoralis minor (page 116). The psoas (page 140), rectus femoris (page 138), and tensor fasciae latae (page 136) can also refer pain here.

Tip: Elevating the head of your bed frame 3 to 3½ inches often stops the swelling in the hands and speeds up recovery.

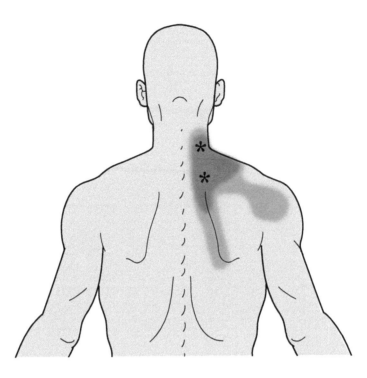

Levator Scapulae

Where it hurts: The crook of your neck, next to your shoulder blade, as well as along the top of the shoulder blade.

You might also be experiencing: Difficulty turning your neck toward the treatment side.

It's often caused by: Whiplash injury, stress, holding your shoulders up around your ears while driving.

Step 1: **Treat the Spine**

- Using a Big Bend Backnobber, Acumasseur, or Thumbby, apply pressure to the deep paraspinal muscles just beside the C3–C5 vertebrae in the middle of the neck.

- Hold the pressure for between 10 and 90 seconds.

Step 2: **Floss the Nerve**

- Do the Scapula Scooper nerve floss (page 75) to floss the dorsal scapular nerve.

Step 3: **Treat the Trigger Points**

- Turn your head toward the treatment side and notice where it pulls or feels tight. That's the spot to target.

- You can reach the corner of your neck, but it's hard to press through the overlying trapezius with your fingers, so I like a Backnobber or Original Worm to get this one. The tender areas will be easy to find.

- Hold the pressure for between 10 and 90 seconds per tender spot.

- You can also use the Backnobber, Acumasseur, or Thumbby in the groove next to your spine to apply pressure to the smaller muscles that restrict the levator's movement.

Step 4: **Gently Move**

- Start in a neutral standing or sitting position with your head in a relaxed but upright position, looking forward.

- Lengthen the muscle by turning your head to the non-treatment side. Return to neutral.

- Shorten the muscle by turning your head toward the treatment side. Return to neutral again.

- Repeat a total of five times.

Other muscles to treat: The scalenes (page 52) and sometimes the biceps (page 80).

Tip: Make sure you're pressing on actual muscle. I've seen many people take a tool and grind into the top of the shoulder blade, mistakenly thinking it was a muscle. A good way to tell if you're in the right spot is to check for "give"—muscles always have some give, while bones shouldn't have any.

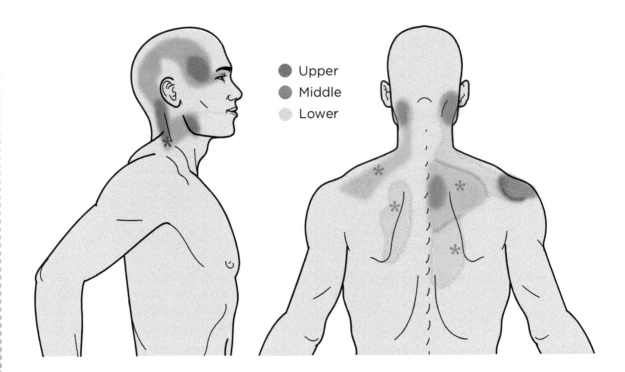

Upper
Middle
Lower

Trapezius

Where it hurts: Trigger points in the *upper* trapezius refer pain up the side of the neck, into the temple, and sometimes into the jaw in a sort of fishhook or question-mark pattern. Trigger points in the *middle* trapezius can cause pain/tingling around the spine and near the top of the shoulder blade. Trigger points in the *lower* trapezius refer pain from the region between the bottom of the shoulder blade and the spine to the upper neck, crook of the neck, and tip of the shoulder.

You might also be experiencing: Temporomandibular joint (TMJ) dysfunction, headaches, hunching your shoulders around your ears.

It's often caused by: Car accidents, stress.

Step 1: Treat the Spine

- Using a Big Bend Backnobber, Acumasseur, or Thumbby, gently apply pressure to the paraspinal muscles just beside the first four vertebrae in the upper neck.

- Hold the pressure for between 10 and 90 seconds.

Step 2: Floss the Nerve

- Do the Shoulder Back, Head Forward nerve floss (page 74) to floss the spinal accessory nerve.

Step 3: Treat the Trigger Points

- Bring your ear toward your shoulder. If you feel a pull, that's the area where the fibers are shortened.

- If the pull is in the upper trapezius, squeeze any tender points between the balls of the Acumasseur. It's simply the best tool for this region, as your fingers will tire quickly. The lower and middle fibers respond best to racquetballs or the Original Worm. Many people love the Backnobber for this region as well.

- Hold the pressure for between 10 and 90 seconds per tender spot.

- Perform the movement a total of five times.

Step 4: Gently Move

Do this as a movement without any breaks. (The movement itself will create the breaks.) The directions may seem complicated, but once you start following them, they'll quickly become clear.

- Stand in a neutral position. Gently press your hands and forearms together in front of you, with your elbows bent, your fingers pointing up, and your thumbs at nose level. This is your starting position.

- To lengthen the muscle, slowly raise your arms toward the ceiling, keeping them pressed together until they naturally begin to separate.

- Let your arms separate and continue to slowly raise them as high as possible, turning your palms forward at full reach.

Continued

- To shorten the muscle, slowly lower your arms, bending your elbows so that they stay pointed downward. Gently squeeze your shoulder blades together as you bring your elbows down.

- Once your elbows are completely lowered, return to the starting position.

- Repeat a total of five times.

Other muscles to treat: The pectorals (pages 114 and 116), serratus anterior (page 122), and sometimes the psoas (page 140), rectus femoris (page 138), and tensor fasciae latae (page 136).

Tip: To treat the upper fibers of the trapezius, try the movement in step 4 of the scalene treatment (page 52).

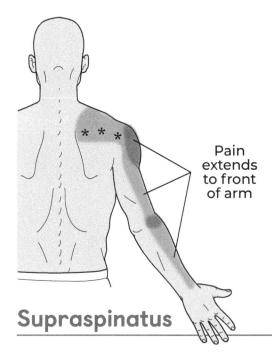

Pain extends to front of arm

Supraspinatus

Where it hurts: This muscle sits on top of the shoulder blade but sends pain to the outside of the shoulder or sometimes down the arm to the elbow.

You might also be experiencing: Snapping or clicking in your shoulder. Some people have trouble lifting their arms to perform daily activities like brushing their teeth, shaving, or combing their hair.

It's often caused by: A tear in the rotator cuff (the group of muscles and tendons around your shoulder joint that lets you lift your arm).

Step 1: Treat the Spine

- Using a Big Bend Backnobber, Acumasseur, or Thumbby, apply pressure to the deep paraspinal muscles right next to the C5 vertebra in the lower neck.

Step 2: Floss the Nerve

- Start in a neutral seated or standing position.

- Exhale as you slowly tilt your head toward the non-treatment shoulder while reaching your treatment arm toward the ceiling. Continue the motion, bending your elbow to bring your hand behind your head.

Continued

- Return the arm to neutral, but keep your head tilted.

- Repeat a total of 10 times.

Step 3: **Treat the Trigger Points**

- Reach your treatment arm behind you and up between your shoulder blades. If you notice any tightness or pulling in the area above your shoulder blade, that's the spot to target.

- Press through the overlying trapezius muscle to reach the supraspinatus. Your fingers can technically do this, but I strongly recommend using a Backnobber, which gives better leverage and saves your hands.

- Hold the pressure for between 10 and 90 seconds per tender spot.

Step 4: **Gently Move**

- Start in a neutral seated or standing position. Hold your treatment arm out to your side with the elbow bent, the palm facing forward, and the fingers together, as if indicating "Stop" or signaling a right turn on a bike. (See illustration on opposite page.)

- Lengthen the muscle by straightening the elbow and reaching up toward the ceiling. Return to neutral.

- Shorten the muscle by lowering the arm while keeping the elbow bent so that your upper arm is flush against your side and your forearm is perpendicular to your body. Keep the fingers together with the palm facing forward.

- Repeat a total of five times.

Other muscles to treat: The infraspinatus (page 62) can sometimes refer pain to the supraspinatus.

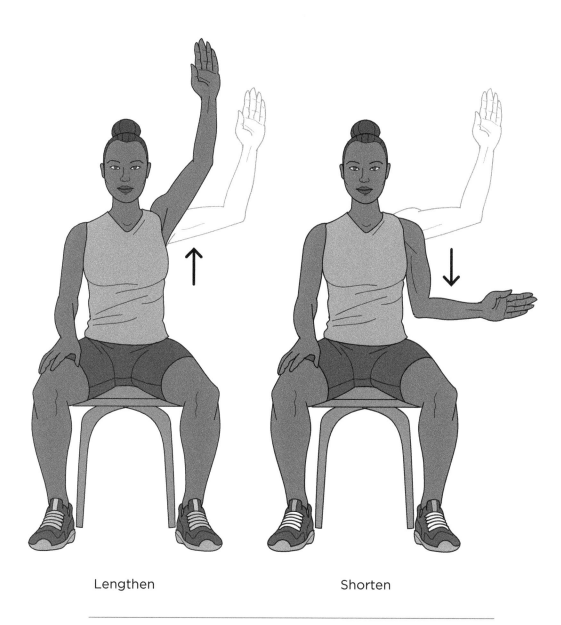

Lengthen   Shorten

Tip: If you can't lift your arm out to the side of your body, see your doctor.
Trigger point therapy will not fix this condition.

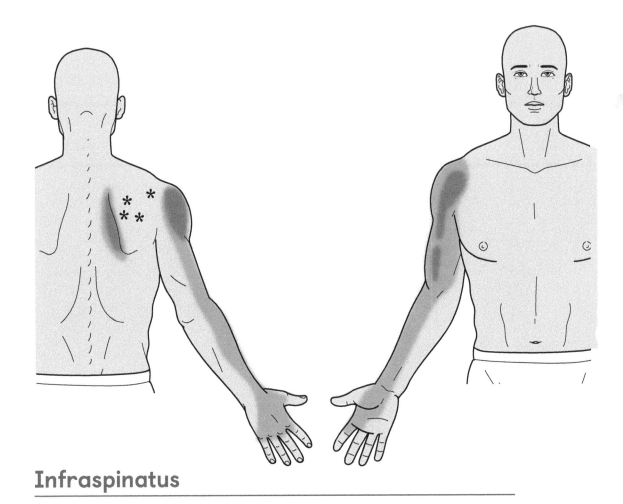

Infraspinatus

Where it hurts: Deep pain in the front of the shoulder that goes down the arm (but skips the elbow) as well as pain beside your shoulder blade.

You might also be experiencing: Difficulty reaching your hand behind your back and up between your shoulder blades. I've also seen many cases of referred numbness and tingling down the arm from this muscle.

It's often caused by: Dislocating your shoulder or experiencing an acute overload, like falling when holding a ski pole or trying to break a fall.

Step 1: **Treat the Spine**

- Using a Big Bend Backnobber, Acumasseur, or Thumbby, apply pressure to the small paraspinal muscles right next to the C5–C6 vertebrae at the bottom of your neck.

Step 2: Floss the Nerve

- Start in a neutral seated or standing position.

- Exhale as you slowly tilt your head toward the non-treatment shoulder while reaching your treatment arm toward the ceiling. Continue the motion, bending your elbow to bring your hand behind your head.

- Return your arm to neutral, but keep your head tilted.

- Repeat a total of 10 times.

Step 3: Treat the Trigger Points

- Reach your treatment arm behind you and up between your shoulder blades. If you notice any tightness or pulling in the back of your shoulder blade, that's the spot to target.

- This spot sits on the back of your shoulder blade and can be reached with a ball, Original Worm, or Backnobber. The spots are very tender and easy to find.

- Hold the pressure for between 10 and 90 seconds per tender spot.

Step 4: Gently Move

The directions for this movement seem complicated at first, but once you start following them, you'll quickly get the gist.

- Start in a neutral seated or standing position.

- Lengthen the muscle by turning your head away from the treatment side and reaching the treatment arm around the back of your head so that your fingers are touching the corner of your mouth (or close to it). Return to neutral.

- Shorten the muscle by putting the treatment arm behind your back and reaching your hand up between your shoulder blades. The back of your hand should be flat against your back with your palm facing outward. Return to neutral.

- Repeat a total of five times.

Other muscles to treat: The supraspinatus (page 59) can sometimes refer pain to the infraspinatus.

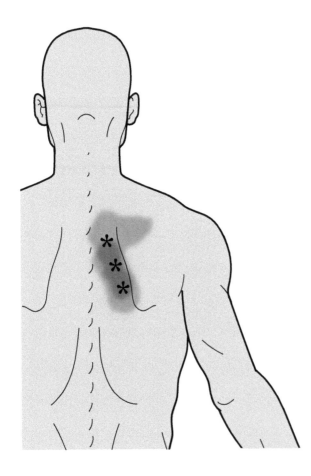

Rhomboids

Where it hurts: Along the inside of your shoulder blade.

You might also be experiencing: Rounded shoulders, carrying your head too far forward.

It's often caused by: Stress—your shoulders instinctively roll forward to protect your vulnerable organs. I often find that dealing with stress is more effective than just muscle treatment.

Step 1: **Treat the Spine**

- Using a Big Bend Backnobber, Acumasseur, or Thumbby, apply pressure to the paraspinal muscles in the lower neck, right next to the C5–C6 vertebrae.

Step 2: Floss the Nerve

- Floss the dorsal scapular nerve with the Scapula Scooper nerve floss (page 75).

Step 3: Treat the Trigger Points

- Press between your shoulder blades, near the blade. You can do this with a tennis ball, Big Bend Backnobber, or the Original Worm.

- Hold the pressure on each tender spot for between 10 and 90 seconds.

Step 4: Gently Move

Do this as a movement without any breaks. (The movement itself will create the breaks.) The directions may seem complicated, but once you start following them, they'll quickly become clear.

- Stand in a neutral position. Gently press your hands and forearms together in front of you with your elbows bent, your fingers pointing up, and your thumbs at nose level. This is your starting position.

- To lengthen the muscle, slowly raise your arms toward the ceiling, keeping them pressed together until they naturally begin to separate.

- Let your arms separate and continue to slowly raise them as high as possible, turning your palms forward at full reach.

- To shorten the muscle, slowly lower your arms, bending your elbows so that they stay pointed downward. Gently squeeze your shoulder blades together as you bring your elbows down.

- Once your elbows are completely lowered, return to the starting position.

- Repeat a total of five times.

Other muscles to treat: The levator scapulae (page 54) and sometimes the pectoralis major (page 114), pectoralis minor (page 116), or serratus anterior (page 122).

Tip: Because this muscle is irritated most by stretching, it would be wise to use a breathing exercise (page 22) and concentrate on practicing the Fidget, Wiggle, and Squirm instructions (page 23).

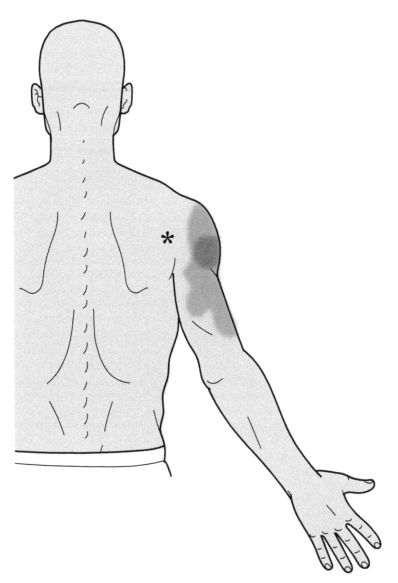

Teres Minor

Where it hurts: Deep in the back of your shoulder.

You might also be experiencing: Pain in the front of your shoulder from related muscles.

It's often caused by: Shoulder trauma.

Step 1: Treat the Spine

- Using a Big Bend Backnobber, Acumasseur, or Thumbby, apply pressure to the paraspinal muscles just beside the C5–C6 vertebrae at the bottom of the neck.

Step 2: Floss the Nerve

- Start in a neutral seated or standing position.

- Exhale as you slowly raise the treatment hand overhead while simultaneously tilting your ear toward the same side. Return to neutral.

- Repeat a total of 10 times.

Step 3: Treat the Trigger Points

- Lie on your treatment side. Bring your treatment arm up straight overhead and roll onto a tennis ball (still lying on your side) so that the ball is at the top of the shoulder blade. This can also be done against a wall with the Original Worm.

- Hold the pressure for between 10 and 90 seconds per tender spot.

Step 4: Gently Move

See page 61 in the supraspinatus entry for illustrations of this movement.

- Start in a neutral seated or standing position. Hold your treatment arm out to your side with the elbow bent, the palm facing forward, and the fingers together, as if indicating "Stop" or signaling a right turn on a bike.

- Lengthen the muscle by straightening the elbow and reaching up toward the ceiling. Return to neutral.

- Shorten the muscle by lowering the arm while keeping the elbow bent so that your upper arm is flush against your side and your forearm is perpendicular to your body. Keep the fingers together with the palm facing forward.

- Repeat a total of five times.

Other muscles to treat: The infraspinatus (page 62) can sometimes refer pain here.

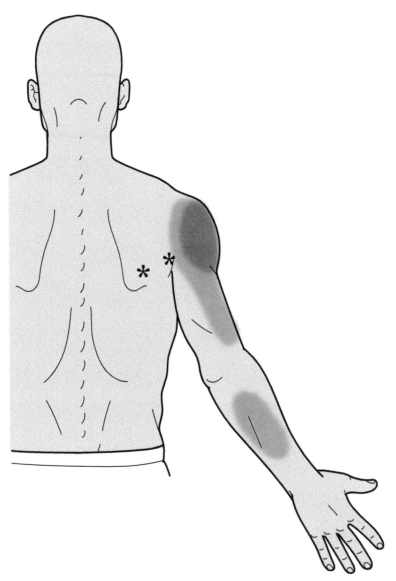

Teres Major

Where it hurts: In the back of the shoulder as well as the back of the arm and forearm. (I once heard Dr. Travell call this "a stupid little muscle.")

You might also be experiencing: Difficulty lifting your arm over your head.

It's often caused by: Strain or trauma on the muscle, as when breaking a fall. Mine really flared when my power steering went out.

Step 1: Treat the Spine

- Using a Big Bend Backnobber, Acumasseur, or Thumbby, apply pressure to the paraspinal muscles next to the C5–C6 vertebrae in the lower neck.

Step 2: Floss the Nerve

- Do the Elbow Bend and Twist nerve floss (page 118) to floss the long thoracic nerve.

Step 3: Treat the Trigger Points

- Point your thumb up and lift your arm behind your head, keeping the elbow straight—when your arm is lifted completely, your straightened elbow should be behind your ear. You'll feel a tightness or pull where the trigger points are restricting this movement.

- You can reach across your body with the non-treatment hand to squeeze this tender spot, but I prefer to lean into it with the Original Worm or squeeze it with the Acumasseur. You can also roll onto a ball on the floor to get it.

- Hold the pressure for between 10 and 90 seconds per tender spot.

Step 4: Gently Move

See page 61 in the supraspinatus entry for illustrations of this movement.

- Start in a neutral seated or standing position. Hold your treatment arm out to your side with the elbow bent, the palm facing forward, and the fingers together, as if indicating "Stop" or signaling a right turn on a bike.

- Lengthen the muscle by straightening the elbow and reaching up toward the ceiling. Return to neutral.

- Shorten the muscle by lowering the arm while keeping the elbow bent so that your upper arm is flush against your side and your forearm is perpendicular to your body. Keep the fingers together with the palm facing forward.

- Repeat a total of five times.

Other muscles to treat: Sometimes the latissimus dorsi (page 119) can refer pain here.

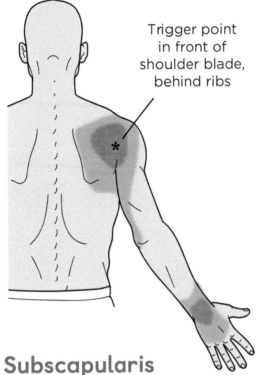

Trigger point
in front of
shoulder blade,
behind ribs

*

Subscapularis

Where it hurts: In the back of your shoulder blade and in a small patch that resembles a watchband on the wrist.

You might also be experiencing: Trouble reaching behind your head, severely restricted shoulder motion ("frozen shoulder").

It's often caused by: Strain on the shoulder from actions like swinging a child around, pitching a ball, or swimming.

Step 1: Treat the Spine

- Using a Big Bend Backnobber, Acumasseur, or Thumbby, apply pressure to the deep paraspinal muscles right next to the C5–C6 vertebrae in the lower neck.

Step 2: Floss the Nerve

- Start in a neutral seated or standing position.

- Make a loose fist with your treatment hand. Bend your elbow and raise that arm to your side until it's level with your shoulder so that it's in an L shape at shoulder level, parallel to the ground, with the knuckles facing forward, almost as if you're about to throw a punch.

- Exhale as you slowly pull your treatment-side elbow and shoulder blade back while simultaneously lowering your ear toward the treatment shoulder.

- Repeat a total of 10 times.

Step 3: Treat the Trigger Points

- From a neutral seated position, lean over so that your treatment hand is dangling down toward the floor.

- Brace your treatment-side elbow on your knee and reach into your armpit with your treatment hand, palm open.

- Use your body weight to apply pressure to any tender spots. Hold the pressure for between 10 and 90 seconds per spot.

Step 4: Gently Move

The directions here seem complicated at first, but once you start following them, they'll quickly become clear.

- Start in a neutral seated or standing position.

- To lengthen the muscle, put the treatment arm behind your back and reach your hand up between your shoulder blades. The back of your hand should be flat against your back with your palm facing outward. Return to neutral.

- To shorten the muscle, turn your head away from the treatment side and reach the treatment arm around the back of your head so that your fingers are touching the corner of your mouth (or close to it). Return to neutral.

- Repeat a total of five times.

Other muscles to treat: The pectoralis major (page 114), teres major (page 68), latissimus dorsi (page 119), deltoid (page 78), and triceps (page 84).

Tip: If you feel numbness or tingling, you may be pressing on your nerve. Move off that spot.

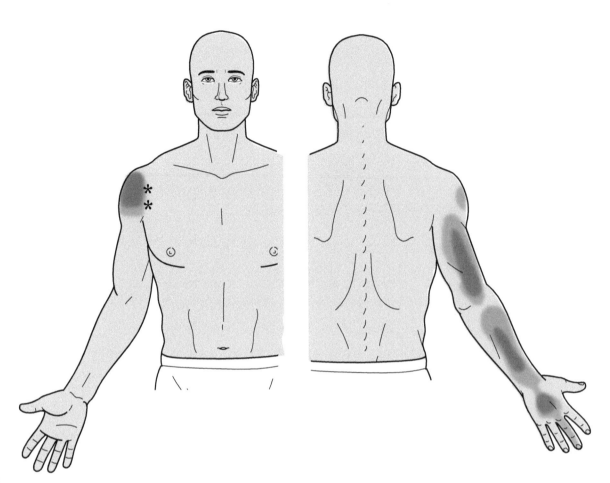

Coracobrachialis

Where it hurts: In the front of the shoulder as well as down the back of the arm into the back of the hand.

You might also be experiencing: Decreased mobility in your shoulder; pain when performing tasks that involve lifting your arm, such as brushing your hair.

It's often caused by: Reaching your arms out in front of you to do heavy work, like lifting.

Step 1: Treat the Spine

- Using a Big Bend Backnobber, Acumasseur, or Thumbby, apply pressure to the deep paraspinal muscles right next to the C5–C6 vertebrae in your lower neck.

Step 2: Floss the Nerve

- Start in a neutral seated or standing position with your treatment arm dangling neutrally at your side and your palm facing your body.

- Keeping the treatment arm at your side, slowly rotate the palm away from your body while simultaneously bringing your ear toward the same shoulder. Exhale as you do so.

- Return to neutral.

- Repeat a total of 10 times.

Step 3: Treat the Trigger Points

- Stand facing a mirror. Wrap your treatment arm behind your head until your fingers are visible on the other side, reaching toward the corner of your mouth. Alternatively, you can wrap your treatment arm behind your back until your fingers are visible on the other side. Either way, you should feel a pull where the trigger point is located.

- Use curved fingers to reach in front of your deltoid (the large muscle covering the top of your shoulder) and under your pectoralis major.

- Press diagonally toward the cap of your shoulder where you felt the pull, probing the front of the shoulder for tender spots.

- Apply and hold pressure for between 10 and 90 seconds per tender spot.

Step 4: Gently Move

- Stand in a neutral position with your arms hanging at your sides.

- Lengthen the muscle by gently reaching your treatment arm straight back behind you (from its lowest point, *not* lifting it overhead). Return to neutral.

- Shorten the muscle by gently lifting your treatment arm in front of you and reaching in the opposite direction so that your arm is at a slight diagonal (so if you raise your right arm, it should be reaching forward and to the left). Return to neutral.

- Repeat a total of five times.

Other muscles to treat: The deltoid (page 78), the pectoralis major (page 114), and occasionally the triceps (page 84).

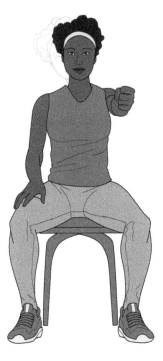

NERVE FLOSS: Shoulder Back, Head Forward

This movement flosses the spinal accessory nerve that supplies the trapezius (page 56) and sternocleidomastoid (page 50) muscles. It's great if you have pain in your neck and head.

Instructions

- Start in a neutral standing or sitting position. Your head should be in a relaxed but upright position, looking forward.

- Make the hand on the treatment side into a soft fist with the thumb lying on top. Keeping your shoulder relaxed, extend that arm straight in front of you so that the bottom of your fist is parallel with the floor.

- Move the treatment-side shoulder back as your head begins to move forward. Keep your neck straight and exhale as you slowly move your head forward and then to the opposite side in a smooth motion.

- Repeat a total of 10 times.

Tip: It helps to practice the two movements separately before putting them together.

NERVE FLOSS: Scapula Scooper

This movement flosses the dorsal scapular nerve in your neck that supplies the rhomboids (page 64) and levator scapulae (page 54). It's helpful if you have pain in your upper back and lower neck.

Instructions

- Start lying on your back in a neutral, relaxed position. (With practice, you can also do it in a neutral standing or sitting position, but lying down is easiest.)

- Exhale as you slowly "scoop" the bottom of your treatment-side shoulder blade inward and upward, as if trying to touch your nose with it.

- At the same time, lean your head toward the treatment side so that your ear slowly lowers toward the shoulder.

- Repeat a total of 10 times.

Tip: It helps to practice the two movements separately before putting them together.

CHAPTER FIVE

Arms and Hands

Trigger points can cause many problems in the arms and hands, and are often a part of other diagnoses that you may have. Learning to work on your own arms can contribute significantly to relieving pain associated with conditions like tennis elbow, carpal tunnel syndrome, and even arthritis. Taking care of the nerves that supply the muscles makes a really big difference in the outcome. The lower neck is the nerve supply for the entire arm, so treating the paraspinal muscles there at the beginning of each session will be important for all the muscles in this chapter.

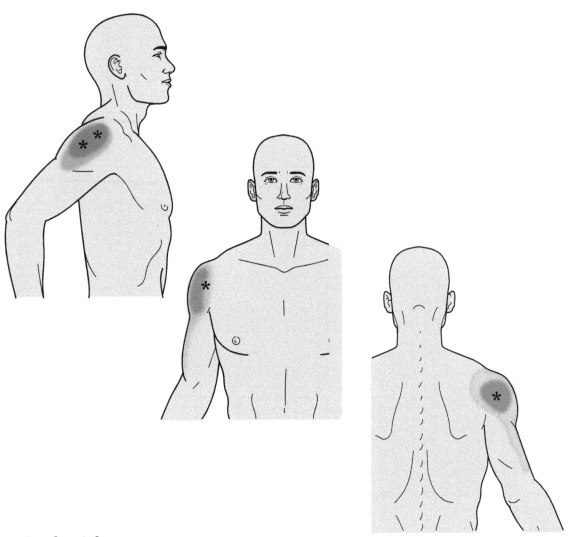

Deltoid

Where it hurts: In the shoulder, most often in the front.

You might also be experiencing: A "catch" when lifting your arm during routine activities like eating or brushing your teeth. The front of the shoulder is often so tight that you're unable to reach your hand behind you between your shoulder blades.

It's often caused by: Trauma or strain to the muscle, such as a fall or recoil from a rifle (people often come to see me with this problem during hunting season).

Step 1: Treat the Spine

- Using a Big Bend Backnobber, Acumasseur, or Thumbby, apply pressure to the paraspinal muscles in the lower neck, right next to the C5–C6 vertebrae.

Step 2: Floss the Nerve

- Floss the axillary nerve on both sides by slowly pressing both shoulders down at the same time, then rolling them in toward the middle at the same time.

- Repeat a total of 10 times.

Step 3: Treat the Trigger Points

- To find the tender spots, probe just below the top of the shoulder, in front and back. For pain on the side of the shoulder, the spots are often located throughout the outside of your upper arm.

- Use a tennis ball or Original Worm to apply pressure.

- Hold the pressure for between 10 and 90 seconds per tender spot.

Step 4: Gently Move

- Start in a neutral seated or standing position. Hold your treatment arm out to your side with the elbow bent, the palm facing forward, and the fingers together, as if indicating "Stop" or signaling a right turn on a bike.

- To lengthen the muscle, keep your arm in that L-shaped position but move it slowly backward. Return to neutral.

- To shorten the muscle, keep your arm in that L-shaped position but slowly move it forward and across your body. Return to neutral.

- Repeat a total of five times.

Other muscles to treat: The infraspinatus (page 62), the scalenes (page 52), and occasionally the coracobrachialis (page 72).

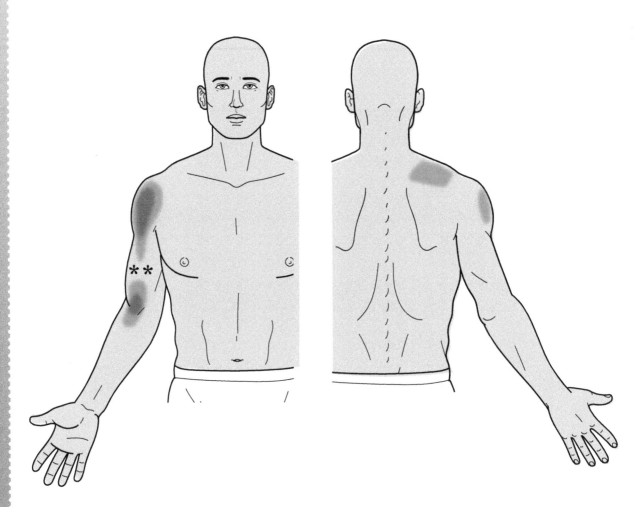

Biceps

Where it hurts: In the front of your elbow and superficially in the shoulder.

You might also be experiencing: Difficulty turning your head to the side, weakness of the arm.

It's often caused by: Heavy lifting.

Step 1: Treat the Spine

- Using a Big Bend Backnobber, Acumasseur, or Thumbby, apply pressure to the paraspinal muscles in the lower neck, right next to the C5–C6 vertebrae.

Step 2: Floss the Nerve

- Start by sitting or standing in a neutral position with your hands at your sides.

- Slowly rotate the treatment-side palm away from your body while simultaneously bringing your ear toward the same shoulder. Exhale as you do so.

- Repeat a total of 10 times.

Step 3: Treat the Trigger Points

- In order to find the trigger points, hold on to a doorframe with your thumb pointed down and turn away from it, noticing where you feel tightness in your biceps.

- Feel for tender spots in the front of the arm about one-third of the way between the elbow and the shoulder.

- Using your fingers or a Thumbby, apply pressure for between 10 and 90 seconds per tender spot.

Step 4: Gently Move

- Sit or stand in a neutral position with your arms relaxed at your sides.

- Lengthen the muscle by opening the palm forward and moving the arm backward behind you while keeping your elbow straight. Return to neutral.

- Shorten the muscle by bending the elbow and raising your open palm toward the same shoulder. Return to neutral again.

- Repeat a total of five times.

Other muscles to treat: Sometimes the infraspinatus (page 62) and brachialis (page 82) can refer pain here.

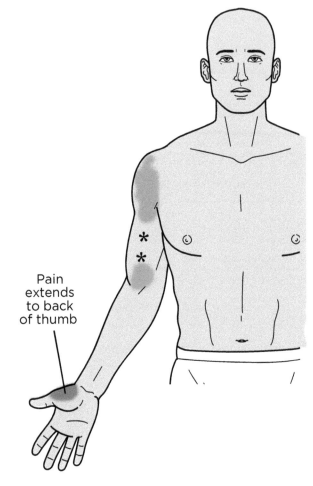

Pain
extends
to back
of thumb

Brachialis

Where it hurts: Intense pain at the base of your thumb with some lesser pain in your upper arm.

You might also be experiencing: When it's really tight, you can't straighten your elbow.

It's often caused by: Keeping the elbow bent for too long during activities like using power tools, playing the guitar, or carrying heavy items.

Step 1: **Treat the Spine**

- Using a Big Bend Backnobber, Acumasseur, or Thumbby, apply pressure to the paraspinal muscles in the lower neck, right next to the C5–C6 vertebrae.

Step 2: **Floss the Nerve**

- Start by sitting or standing in a neutral position with your hands at your sides.

- Keeping your hands at your sides, open the palm and slowly turn it so that it faces forward as you straighten the elbow on the treatment side. At the same time, tilt your ear toward the treatment shoulder.

- Repeat a total of 10 times.

Step 3: **Treat the Trigger Points**

- Reach your non-treatment arm across your body to the treatment arm.

- Relax the treatment arm and gently move the bicep away from the body to get to the underlying brachialis.

- Using a Thumbby, apply pressure to any tender spots, holding for between 10 and 90 seconds per spot.

Step 4: **Gently Move**

- Sit or stand in a neutral position.

- Lengthen the muscle by raising your treatment arm, bending the elbow, and reaching behind you, as if you were trying to scratch between your shoulder blades. Return to neutral.

- Shorten the muscle by straightening the elbow and reaching backward so that your arm is extended behind you (from its lowest point, *not* overhead). Return to neutral again.

- Repeat a total of five times.

Other muscles to treat: The biceps (page 80) and triceps (page 84) can sometimes refer pain here.

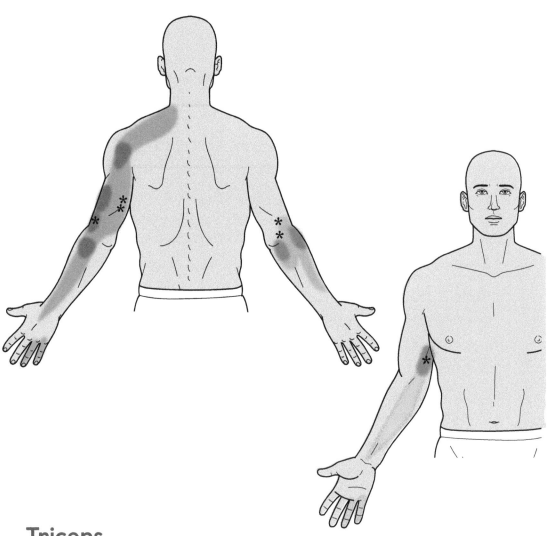

Triceps

Where it hurts: In the back of the shoulder, arm, and elbow.

You might also be experiencing: Numbness and tingling in the back of your arm, "tennis elbow," pain when playing golf or tennis. You'll find that you can't bend the elbow and point it toward the ceiling so that it's stretched behind your ear.

It's often caused by: Excessive use of crutches, too many push-ups.

Step 1: Treat the Spine

- Using the Big Bend Backnobber or a similar tool, apply pressure to the paraspinal muscles in the lowest part of the neck, right next to the C7–T1 vertebrae.

Step 2: Floss the Nerve

- Do the Tip Your Server nerve floss (page 104) to floss the radial nerve.

Step 3: Treat the Trigger Points

- To find the tender spots, try to bend your treatment-side elbow and reach overhead and behind you, as if you were going to scratch between your shoulder blades. The place where you feel a pull in your upper arm is where you'll find the trigger point(s).

- Lay your arm, palm facing upward, on a table.

- Place a tennis ball between the table and the part of your upper arm where you felt trigger points.

- Press down on any tender spots. The weight of your arm provides all the pressure you need.

- Hold the pressure for between 10 and 90 seconds per tender spot.

Step 4: Gently Move

- Sit or stand in a neutral position with your arms relaxed at your sides.

- Lengthen the muscle by raising your treatment arm, bending the elbow, and reaching up and behind you, as if you were trying to scratch between your shoulder blades. Return to neutral.

- Shorten the muscle by straightening the elbow and reaching backward so that your arm is extended behind you (with your palm toward the ground). Return to neutral again.

- Repeat a total of five times.

Other muscles to treat: Sometimes the coracobrachialis (page 72) can refer pain here.

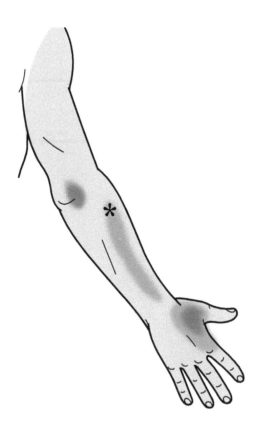

Brachioradialis

Where it hurts: The outside of your elbow and the fleshy area between your thumb and index finger. (A similar pain pattern occurs with trigger points in the supinator.)

You might also be experiencing: A weak grip. The cluster of symptoms people with these trigger points experience is often called "tennis elbow."

It's often caused by: Keeping the elbow and wrist straight during a backhand when playing tennis, scraping the ice from a windshield, or doing a lot of handshaking (in a receiving line, for example).

Step 1: Treat the Spine

- Using a Big Bend Backnobber, Acumasseur, or Thumbby, apply pressure to the paraspinal muscles in the lower neck, right next to the C5–C6 vertebrae.

Step 2: Floss the Nerve

- Floss the radial nerve with the Tip Your Server nerve floss (page 104).

Step 3: Treat the Trigger Points

- Bend your elbow, pointing your thumb up and tensing the uppermost part of your forearm. Use your fingers to probe the upper half of your forearm for tender spots—there are often a number of them.

- Tender spots can be trapped and gently squeezed using the Acumasseur or your fingers.

- Hold the gentle squeeze for between 10 and 90 seconds per tender spot.

Step 4: Gently Move

- Start by standing in a neutral position with your arms relaxed at your sides.

- On the treatment side, press your shoulder downward without moving your head or torso.

- To lengthen the muscle, cup your palm as you gently flex your wrist so that your palm is facing upward and rotate it back, kind of like you're slipping a tip to your server.

- Shorten the muscle by relaxing your shoulder and opening your palm so that it faces forward. Return to center again.

- Repeat a total of five times.

Other muscles to treat: Sometimes the supinator (page 88) and/or wrist extensors (page 90) can refer pain here.

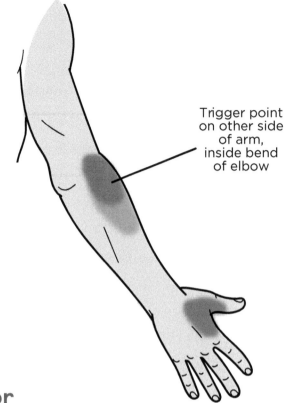

Trigger point
on other side
of arm,
inside bend
of elbow

Supinator

Where it hurts: The outside of the elbow and the fleshy area between your thumb and forefinger. (A similar pain pattern occurs with trigger points in the brachioradialis.)

You might also be experiencing: Pain when carrying a bag with the elbow open. You might struggle with some ranges of motion, like bending your elbow and turning your palm so that it faces toward the floor.

It's often caused by: Strain on your forearms, such as when opening a tight jar or walking a large dog.

Step 1: **Treat the Spine**

- Using a Big Bend Backnobber, Acumasseur, or Thumbby, apply pressure to the paraspinal muscles in the lower neck, right next to the C5–C7 vertebrae.

Step 2: **Floss the Nerve**

- Floss the radial nerve with the Tip Your Server nerve floss (page 104).

Step 3: **Treat the Trigger Points**

- Grasp the overlying brachioradialis by bending the elbow with your hand held sideways and your thumb pointing up. As soon as the palm turns up, the supinator is right there. Resting your arm on a table while you do this can be helpful.

- Turn the palm upward. Use a Thumbby to press down on the inside of the brachioradialis, just below the elbow.

- Hold the pressure for between 10 and 90 seconds per tender spot.

Step 4: **Gently Move**

- Sit or stand in a neutral position with your arms at your sides.

- Lengthen the muscle by twisting the treatment arm so that your palm faces outward. Return to center.

- Shorten the muscle by twisting your arm so that the palm faces your body. Return to center again.

- Repeat a total of five times.

Other muscles to treat: The brachioradialis (page 86) and wrist extensors (page 90).

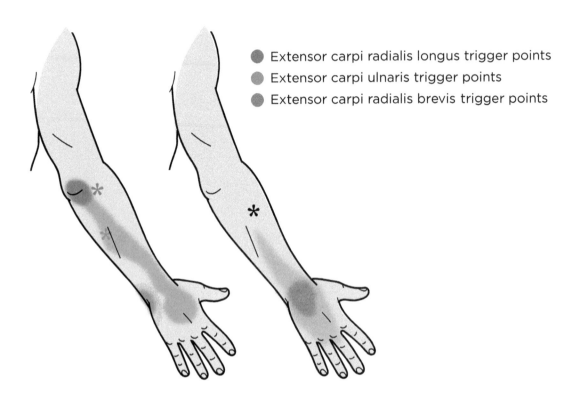

- ● Extensor carpi radialis longus trigger points
- ● Extensor carpi ulnaris trigger points
- ● Extensor carpi radialis brevis trigger points

Wrist Extensors
Extensor Carpi Radialis Longus, Extensor Carpi Radialis Brevis, Extensor Carpi Ulnaris

Where it hurts: Your elbow and the back of your wrist.

You might also be experiencing: Pain and weakness during activities that involve wrist motion, like shaking hands, opening a tight jar, or turning a doorknob.

It's often caused by: Using hand tools or squeezing a ball to test strength.

Step 1: Treat the Spine

- Using a Big Bend Backnobber, Acumasseur, or Thumbby, apply pressure to the paraspinal muscles in the very lowest part of your neck, right next to the C6–T1 vertebrae.

Step 2: Floss the Nerve

- Floss the radial nerve with the Tip Your Server nerve floss (page 104).

Step 3: Treat the Trigger Points

- In order to find the tender spots, put your arm in front of you with the palm down. Gently pull the hand down to bend the wrist, paying attention to any areas where you feel a pull.

- Place your palm down on the table with your elbow bent and probe just below the elbow for tender spots where you felt the pull.

- Press the tender spots with a Thumbby, or bend your elbow and press against a tennis ball held between the back of your forearm and the wall.

- Hold the pressure for between 10 and 90 seconds per tender spot.

Step 4: Gently Move

- Sit or stand in a neutral position with your arms relaxed at your sides.

- To lengthen the muscle, raise your arm directly in front of you so it forms a 90-degree angle with your body, then bend your wrist downward so that your fingers point toward the floor and your palm faces you. Return to neutral.

- Shorten the muscle by raising your arm with your wrist facing the ceiling and then flexing your wrist back so that your fingers point to the floor and your palm faces away from you. Return to neutral again.

- Repeat a total of five times.

Other muscles to treat: The supinator (page 88) and scalenes (page 52).

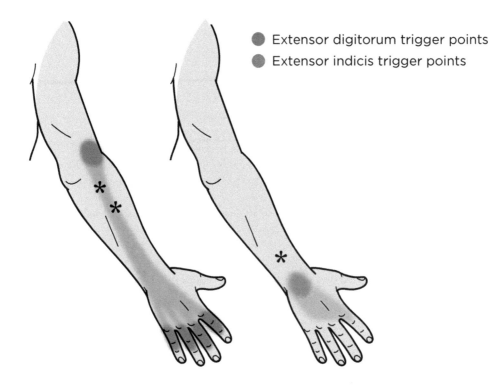

● Extensor digitorum trigger points
● Extensor indicis trigger points

Finger Extensors
Extensor Digitorum, Extensor Indicis

Where it hurts: Primarily the back of the forearm and fingers.

You might also be experiencing: Elbow pain and finger stiffness.

It's often caused by: Playing an instrument or working with tools for long periods.

Step 1: Treat the Spine

- Using a Big Bend Backnobber, Acumasseur, or Thumbby, apply pressure to the paraspinal muscles in the very lowest part of your neck, right next to the C6–T1 vertebrae.

Step 2: Floss the Nerve

- Floss the radial nerve with the Tip Your Server nerve floss (page 104).

Step 3: Treat the Trigger Points

- Place your arm on a table or pillow with the palm up and the elbow bent. Probe the upper forearm for tender spots.

- Use the Thumbby to press any tender spots in the upper forearm, or bend the elbow and apply pressure with a tennis ball or Original Worm held between your forearm and a wall.

- Hold the pressure for between 10 and 90 seconds per tender spot.

Step 4: Gently Move

- Sit or stand in a neutral position with your arms relaxed at your sides.

- To lengthen the muscle, keep your arm at your side and gently bend your wrist with your fingers extended so that your palm is facing up and your fingers point behind you. Return to neutral.

- To shorten the muscle, gently bend your wrist the opposite way so that your palm is facing down and your fingers point forward. Return to neutral again.

- Repeat a total of five times.

Other muscles to treat: The wrist extensors (page 90) as well as, less frequently, the brachioradialis (page 86), finger flexors (page 98), and wrist flexors (page 96).

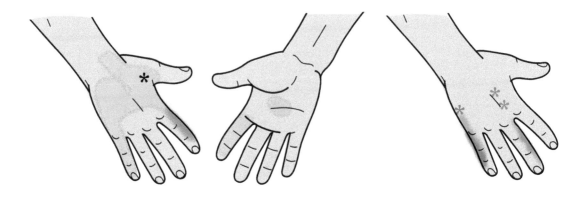

● First dorsal interosseus trigger points
● Abductor digiti minimi trigger points
● Second dorsal interosseus trigger points

Dorsal Interossei

Where it hurts: Primarily along the side(s) of the affected finger(s), sometimes in the palm and back of the hand.

You might also be experiencing: Difficulty with fine-motor activities, like fastening buttons, writing with a pen, and grasping.

It's often caused by: Using a repetitive "pincer grip," as in sewing or detailed mechanical work.

Step 1: **Treat the Spine**

- Using a Big Bend Backnobber, Acumasseur, or Thumbby, apply pressure to the paraspinal muscles in the very lowest part of your neck, right next to the C7–T1 vertebrae.

Step 2: **Floss the Nerve**

- Floss the radial nerve supply with the Tip Your Server nerve floss (page 104).

Step 3: **Treat the Trigger Points**

- Lift and separate the bones in the hand to expose the muscles on the side.

- Use your non-treatment fingers to apply gentle pressure to any tender areas.

- Hold the pressure for between 10 and 90 seconds per tender spot.

Step 4: **Gently Move**

- There is no Swedish movement for these muscles.

Other muscles to treat: It can sometimes be helpful to treat the wrist flexors (page 96), finger flexors (page 98), wrist extensors (page 90), and finger extensors (page 92).

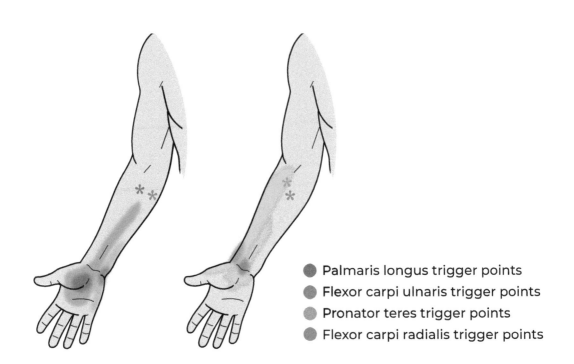

● Palmaris longus trigger points
● Flexor carpi ulnaris trigger points
● Pronator teres trigger points
● Flexor carpi radialis trigger points

Wrist Flexors
Flexor Carpi Ulnaris, Flexor Carpi Radialis, Palmaris Longus, Pronator Teres

Where it hurts: The palm and/or palm side of the wrist and forearm.

You might also be experiencing: Difficulty using objects that require fine-motor skills, like scissors or curlers.

It's often caused by: An elbow that has been broken in the past, grasping objects like a steering wheel or hand tools too tightly.

Step 1: Treat the Spine

- Using the Big Bend Backnobber or a similar tool, apply pressure to the paraspinal muscles in the very lowest part of your neck, right next to the C6–T1 vertebrae.

Step 2: Floss the Nerve

- Floss the nerve supply with the Tunnel Tamer nerve floss (page 106) or the Eye Piece nerve floss (page 105)—whichever seems to work better for you.

Step 3: Treat the Trigger Points

- To locate the trigger points, place your treatment-side forearm on a table with your palm up. Then feel for tension or tenderness with these specific tests.
  - *For the pronator teres:* Turn the forearm inward so your palm is facing toward your body rather than up. Return to neutral.
  - *For the flexor carpi radialis:* Keeping the rest of your hand still, move your wrist toward the thumb side. Return to neutral.
  - *For the palmaris longus:* Cup your hand. Return to neutral.
  - *For the flexor carpi ulnaris:* Keeping the rest of your hand still, move your wrist toward the pinky side. Return to neutral.

- Use the Thumbby to apply pressure to any tender spots you find during the process, holding the pressure for between 10 and 90 seconds per tender spot.

Step 4: Gently Move

- Sit or stand in a neutral position with your treatment arm straight out in front of you.

- To lengthen the muscle, turn your palm upward and gently bend your wrist with your fingers extended so that your fingers point down. Return to neutral.

- To shorten the muscle, turn your palm downward with your fingers pointing forward and gently bend your wrist toward the floor. Return to neutral again.

- Repeat a total of five times.

Other muscles to treat: The wrist extensors (page 90), scalenes (page 52), and pectoralis minor (page 116).

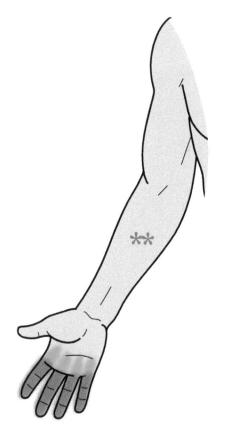

Finger Flexors
Flexor Digitorum Superficialis, Flexor Digitorum Profundus

Where it hurts: Individual fingers.

You might also be experiencing: Difficulty with fine-motor activities that involve gripping, such as using scissors or holding the steering wheel.

It's often caused by: Prolonged gripping.

Step 1: Treat the Spine

- Using the Big Bend Backnobber or a similar tool, apply pressure to the paraspinal muscles in the very lowest part of your neck, right next to the C7–T1 vertebrae.

Step 2: Floss the Nerve

- Floss the nerve supply with the Tunnel Tamer nerve floss (page 106) or the Eye Piece nerve floss (page 105)—whichever seems to work better for you.

Step 3: Treat the Trigger Points

- With your elbow straight, use your non-treatment hand to pull back the individual fingers on your treatment hand. Then try it again with your elbow bent. One or both actions should let you feel where the tight areas are. Mark them with a pen.

- With your elbow bent, rest your forearm on a table, palm up.

- Use a Thumbby to apply pressure where you made pen marks, holding for between 10 and 90 seconds per tender spot.

Step 4: Gently Move

- Sit or stand in a neutral position with your arms relaxed at your sides.

- To lengthen the muscles, keep your arms at your side and gently bend your treatment wrist with your fingers extended so that your palm is facing up and your fingers point behind you. Return to neutral.

- To shorten the muscles, gently bend your wrist the opposite way so that your palm is facing down and your fingers point forward. Return to neutral again.

- Repeat a total of five times.

Other muscles to treat: It can help to treat the wrist flexors (page 96), wrist extensors (page 90), scalenes (page 52), and pectoralis minor (page 116).

Tip: These muscles are deep. Treat the overlying wrist flexors first.

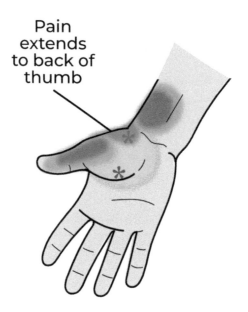

Pain
extends
to back of
thumb

🔘 Opponens pollicis trigger points
🔘 Adductor pollicis trigger points

Adductor/Opponens Pollicis

Where it hurts: The thumb as well as the bottom of the wrist on the same side.

You might also be experiencing: Difficulty with fine-motor activities, like fastening buttons, holding a pen, or writing.

It's often caused by: Using the thumb to massage, weeding the garden, and general overuse of the thumb.

Step 1: Treat the Spine

- Using the Big Bend Backnobber or a similar tool, apply pressure to the paraspinal muscles in the very lowest part of your neck, right next to the C7–T1 vertebrae.

Step 2: Floss the Nerve

- Floss the median nerve with the Tunnel Tamer nerve floss (page 106).

Step 3: Treat the Trigger Points

- Using the Thumbby, apply pressure to any tender areas between the bottom of the thumb and the end of the wrist, and between the base of the thumb and the middle of your hand.

- Hold the pressure on each spot for between 10 and 90 seconds.

Step 4: Gently Move

- Sit or stand in a neutral position with your arms relaxed at your sides.

- Lengthen the muscle by spreading your fingers and opening your hand wide on the treatment side. Return to neutral.

- Shorten the muscle by making a soft fist. Return to neutral.

- Repeat a total of five times.

Other muscles to treat: The scalenes (page 52) and pectoralis minor (page 116) as well as, less frequently, the brachioradialis (page 86), supinator (page 88), wrist flexors (page 96), and finger flexors (page 98).

Tip: Spare your thumbs and use one of the tools recommended in this book to apply pressure to these trigger points!

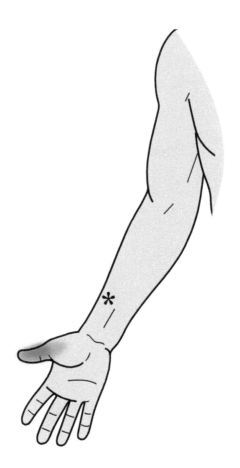

Flexor Pollicis Longus

Where it hurts: The tip of your thumb.

You might also be experiencing: Difficulty with fine-motor activities, like using scissors or holding the steering wheel.

It's often caused by: Prolonged gripping.

Step 1: **Treat the Spine**

- Using the Big Bend Backnobber or a similar tool, apply pressure to the paraspinal muscles in the very lowest part of your neck, right next to the C7–T1 vertebrae.

Step 2: **Floss the Nerve**

- Floss the median nerve with the Tunnel Tamer nerve floss (page 106).

Step 3: **Treat the Trigger Points**

- You can feel where there is tightness by pulling your thumb back.

- Press the tender area where you felt the pull with the Thumbby.

- Hold the pressure for between 10 and 90 seconds per tender spot.

Step 4: **Gently Move**

- Sit or stand in a neutral position with your forearms on a flat surface and your thumb raised so that it's pointing at the ceiling.

- Lengthen the muscle by pulling the thumb back, almost as if you're making a "hitchhiker" motion. Return to neutral.

- Shorten the muscle by moving the thumb forward and down, toward the palm. Return to neutral again.

- Repeat a total of five times.

Other muscles to treat: The adductor/opponens pollicis (page 100) as well as, less frequently, the wrist flexors (page 96), wrist extensors (page 90), scalenes (page 52), and pectoralis minor (page 116).

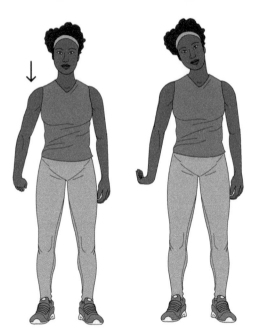

NERVE FLOSS: Tip Your Server

This movement flosses the radial nerve, which supplies
a number of muscles in your arm, including the triceps
(page 84) and the wrist extensors (page 90). The flossing
movement calms the nerve and often relaxes the muscles.

Instructions

- Start by standing in a neutral position with your arms relaxed at
  your sides.

- On the treatment side, press your shoulder downward without moving
  your head or torso.

- Keeping your palm flat and your fingers straight, flex your hand so that
  your palm is facing upward with your fingers pointing back behind you.

- Exhale as you slowly tilt your ear toward the treatment-side shoulder
  while simultaneously rotating your wrist so that your hand is still palm
  up but with your fingers pointing away from your body—almost as
  if you were slipping a tip to a waiter or waitress. Your fingers will
  naturally curl into a sort of J shape as you do so.

- Repeat a total of 10 times.

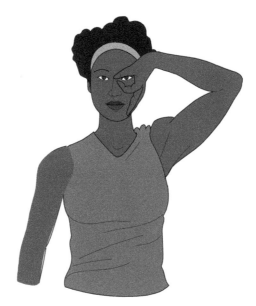

NERVE FLOSS: Eye Piece

This movement flosses the ulnar nerve, which runs to a number of muscles in your forearm and fingers, including certain wrist flexors (page 96) and finger flexors (page 98). (The ulnar nerve is also what hurts when you hit your funny bone.) The flossing movement calms the nerve and often relaxes the muscles.

Instructions

- With your hand in front of your chest, touch your thumb and index finger together, with your other three fingers pointing upward so that you're making an "A-OK" sign.

- Raise your hand to your eye, rotating your wrist toward your body as you do so, so that the A-OK sign is upside down and you're looking through the circle created by your thumb and index finger, with your other three fingers resting on the side of your face below.

- Do the movement slowly as you exhale.

- Repeat a total of 10 times.

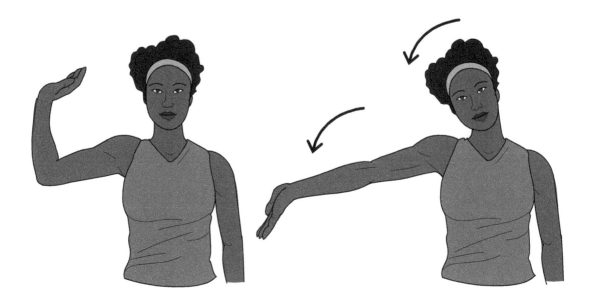

NERVE FLOSS: Tunnel Tamer

This movement flosses the median nerve, which supplies a number of muscles in your arm, including wrist flexors (page 96) and finger flexors (page 98). The flossing movement calms the nerve and often relaxes the muscles.

Instructions

• Start by sitting or standing in a neutral position with your shoulders relaxed and your arms at your sides.

• Bring your arm out to your side with your elbow bent, your forearm parallel to your body, and your wrist flexed. Your palm should be facing upward, and your fingers should be pointing toward your temple.

• Keeping your wrist flexed, straighten your elbow and slightly rotate your forearm so that, by the time your elbow is fully extended, your palm will be facing away from you.

• At the same time, bend the neck to the same side.

• Repeat a total of 10 times.

CHAPTER SIX

Chest, Back, and Abdomen

If you have any type of pain, it is highly likely that you'll find a muscle related to it in this chapter. The paraspinals are really important—they control the nerve supply to pretty much every muscle, and working with them is usually part of a good treatment plan. Trigger points in the abdominal muscles are also related to a host of different types of pain, even counterintuitive ones like heartburn and bowel issues. It's important, however, to err on the side of safety. Abdominal pain and chest pain can be signs of serious non-myofascial issues like ulcers or even heart problems. Before you begin trying these techniques, please consult with your doctor to rule out any other causes for your abdominal or chest pain.

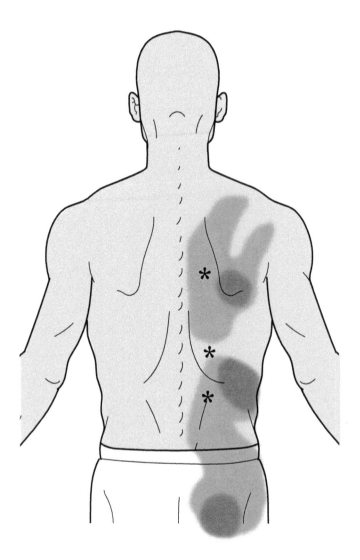

Superficial Paraspinals

Where it hurts: Primarily in the back beside the spine. Pain can also extend into the buttock region.

You might also be experiencing: Restricted ability to move the back.

It's often caused by: Physical trauma, bending and twisting activities, and any problem with normal walking.

Step 1: **Treat the Spine**

- Since you're already targeting the paraspinals, there's no additional spine treatment.

Step 2: **Floss the Nerve**

- Perform the Slumping for Health nerve floss (page 132), or do the Swedish movement in step 4 below a total of 10 times.

Step 3: **Treat the Trigger Points**

- Start by slowly lowering your head and rolling your spine down, as you might when reaching for your toes. You'll feel areas of tightness near the spine as several spinal segments move at once.

- Use a racquetball, tennis ball, or Original Worm to seek out tender points in the tight areas near the spine—but not directly in the gutter next to the bones of the spine. (I prefer the racquetball over the ribs and the tennis ball in the lower back.)

- Apply pressure to any tender spots and hold for 10 to 90 seconds.

Step 4: **Gently Move**

- Start by sitting on the floor with your knees bent, the soles of your feet on the floor, and your spine straight. Put your hands around your legs just below the knees.

- Lengthen the muscle by gently curving your back away from your legs. Return to neutral.

- Shorten the muscle by gently arching your back the opposite way, leaning your belly forward and your head back. Return to neutral.

- Repeat a total of five times.

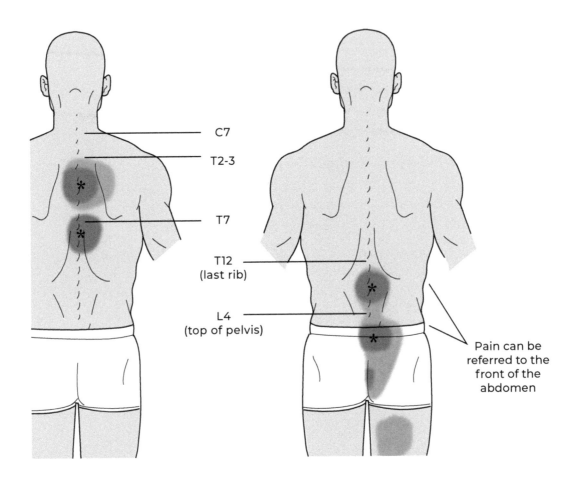

C7

T2-3

T7

T12
(last rib)

L4
(top of pelvis)

Pain can be
referred to the
front of the
abdomen

Deep Paraspinals

Where it hurts: Almost directly on the spine, and possibly shooting around to the front of the body. You might notice pain as you turn to either side, or on both sides.

You might also be experiencing: Restricted ability to move the back.

It's often caused by: Physical trauma, bending and twisting activities, and any problem with normal walking. Sitting for long periods can be brutal as well.

Step 1: Treat the Spine

- Since you're already targeting the paraspinals, there's no additional spine treatment.

Step 2: Floss the Nerve

- Perform the Slumping for Health nerve floss (page 132), or do the Swedish movement in step 4 a total of 10 times.

Step 3: Treat the Trigger Points

- Slowly lower the head and roll the spine down, as you might when reaching for your toes. You'll feel areas of tightness near the spine as several spinal segments move at once.

- Using the Big Bend Backnobber, press the tender spots in the gutter just beside the bony spine. Don't press on the bone itself.

- Hold the pressure for between 10 and 90 seconds per tender spot.

Step 4: Gently Move

- Start by sitting on the floor with your knees bent, the soles of your feet on the floor, and your spine straight. Put your hands around your legs just below the knees.

- Lengthen the muscle by gently curving your back away from your legs. Return to neutral.

- Shorten the muscle by gently arching your back the opposite way, leaning your belly forward and your head back. Return to neutral.

- Repeat a total of five times.

Other muscles to treat: The superficial paraspinals (page 110) as well as, less frequently, the iliopsoas (page 140), tensor fasciae latae (page 136), rectus femoris (page 138), pectoralis major (page 114), pectoralis minor (page 116), and serratus anterior (page 122).

Tip: This and the suboccipitals are the best places to start treatment for any trigger point problem. They help calm the entire nervous system.

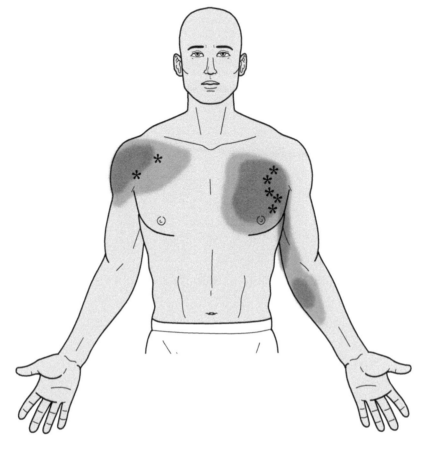

Pectoralis Major

Where it hurts: In your chest and/or the front of your shoulder.

You might also be experiencing: You or others might complain about your posture. You may notice that your shoulders don't touch the ground when you lie down on your back.

It's often caused by: Stress! It makes your shoulders roll forward. You might also spend too much time sitting at a computer or driving with your shoulders slumped.

Step 1: **Treat the Spine**

- Using the Big Bend Backnobber or a similar tool, apply pressure to the paraspinal muscles in the very lowest part of your neck, right next to the C7-T1 vertebrae.

Step 2: Floss the Nerve

- Perform the Slumping for Health (page 132) and Doorway Step (page 133) nerve flosses.

Step 3: Treat the Trigger Points

- Press any tender spots below the collarbone in the chest with a tennis ball, Thumbby, or Original Worm.

- Hold the pressure for between 10 and 90 seconds per tender spot.

Step 4: Gently Move

The directions for this movement seem complicated at first, but once you start following them, you'll quickly get the gist.

- Stand in a neutral position. Gently press your hands and forearms together in front of you with your elbows bent, your fingers pointing up, and your thumbs at nose level. This is your starting position.

- To lengthen the muscle, slowly raise your arms toward the ceiling, keeping them pressed together until they naturally begin to separate.

- Let your arms separate and continue to slowly raise them as high as possible, turning your palms forward at full reach.

- To shorten the muscle, slowly lower your arms, bending your elbows so that they stay pointed downward. Gently squeeze your shoulder blades together as you bring your elbows down.

- Once your elbows are completely lowered, return to the starting position.

- Repeat a total of five times.

Other muscles to treat: The pectoralis minor (page 116), serratus anterior (page 122), superficial paraspinals (page 110), and deep paraspinals (page 112). Sometimes it also helps to treat the iliopsoas (page 140), tensor fasciae latae (page 136), and rectus femoris (page 138).

Tip: If you're experiencing chest pain, it's essential to discuss it with your doctor and determine its cause. Don't perform trigger point therapy until you've established that it's a myofascial issue, not a heart problem.

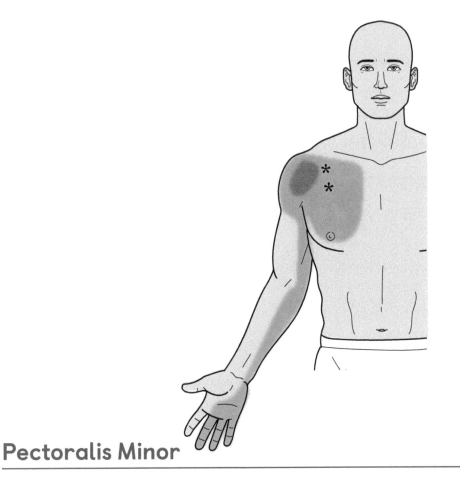

Pectoralis Minor

Where it hurts: In the front of your shoulder and chest, down the inside of your arm.

You might also be experiencing: Numbness and tingling down the arm.

It's often caused by: Stress! It makes your shoulders roll forward. You might also spend too much time sitting at a computer or driving with your shoulders slumped.

Step 1: Treat the Spine

- Using a Big Bend Backnobber, Acumasseur, or Thumbby, apply pressure to the paraspinal muscles in the lower neck and just beside the top of your shoulder blade (near the C7–T1 vertebrae).

Step 2: Floss the Nerve

- Perform the Slumping for Health (page 132) and Doorway Step (page 133) nerve flosses.

Step 3: Treat the Trigger Points

- Press any tender spots below the collarbone in the chest with a tennis ball, Thumbby, or Original Worm. Because you can't move the overlying pectoralis major aside, you will be gently pressing down through it to the pectoralis minor underneath.

- Hold the pressure for between 10 and 90 seconds per tender spot.

Step 4: Gently Move

The directions for this movement seem complicated at first, but once you start following them, you'll quickly get the gist.

- Stand in a neutral position. Gently press your hands and forearms together in front of you with your elbows bent, your fingers pointing up, and your thumbs at nose level. This is your starting position.

- To lengthen the muscle, slowly raise your arms toward the ceiling, keeping them pressed together until they naturally begin to separate.

- Let your arms separate and continue to slowly raise them as high as possible, turning your palms forward at full reach.

- To shorten the muscle, slowly lower your arms, bending your elbows so that they stay pointed downward. Gently squeeze your shoulder blades together as you bring your elbows down.

- Once your elbows are completely lowered, return to the starting position.

- Repeat a total of five times.

Other muscles to treat: The pectoralis major (page 114), serratus anterior (page 122), and superficial paraspinals (page 110). Sometimes it's helpful to treat the iliopsoas (page 140), tensor fasciae latae (page 136), and rectus femoris (page 138).

Tip: If you're experiencing chest pain, it's essential to discuss it with your doctor and determine its cause. Don't perform trigger point therapy until you've established that it's a muscular issue, not a heart problem.

NERVE FLOSS: Elbow Bend and Twist

This movement flosses the long thoracic nerve that supplies the serratus anterior muscles spanning your upper ribs (page 122). The flossing movement calms the nerve and often relaxes the muscle, which can also benefit other muscles it's connected to.

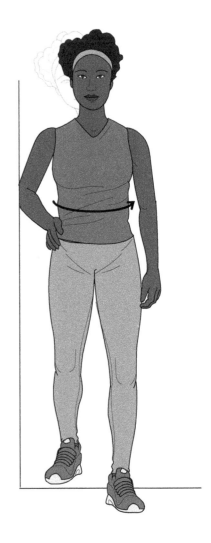

Instructions

• Stand with your treatment-side hand on your hip and the outside of that elbow against a doorframe or wall. Take a step forward with the non-treatment foot so that the treatment foot is back and the non-treatment foot is forward.

• Inhale as you slowly and gently twist your whole torso away from the doorframe while dropping your ear down toward your shoulder on the treatment side. Stop when you feel a gentle pull.

• Exhale as you slowly return to the starting position. Don't rush—this movement should be performed slowly.

• Repeat a total of 10 times.

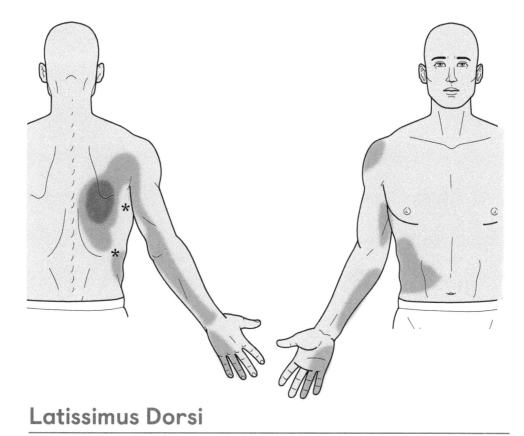

Latissimus Dorsi

Where it hurts: At the bottom of your shoulder blades and sometimes down the pinky side of your arm.

You might also be experiencing: Pain when using your hands to press down when getting out of a chair or when wearing a tight bra.

It's often caused by: Motions like throwing a baseball or pulling a rope. Mine was hurt by trying to break a fall when I was struck by a car while riding my bike.

Continued

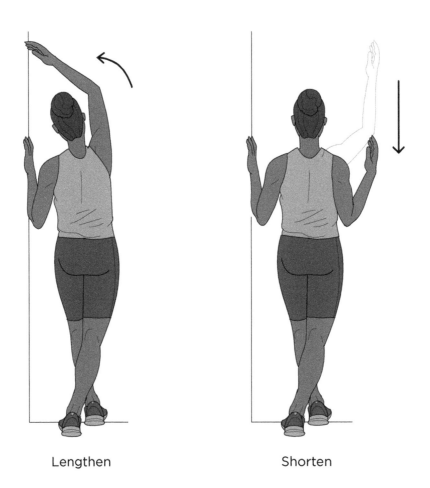

Lengthen   Shorten

Step 1: **Treat the Spine**

- Using a Big Bend Backnobber, Acumasseur, or Thumbby, apply pressure to the paraspinal muscles in the very lowest part of your neck, right next to the C6–T1 vertebrae.

Step 2: **Floss the Nerve**

- Floss the long thoracic nerve with the Elbow Bend and Twist nerve floss (page 118).

Step 3: Treat the Trigger Points

- Start by letting your arm hang by your side and then bringing the hand up in an arc over your head with a straight elbow until the elbow is behind the ear. Any tightness you feel in your middle to lower back is a good place to look for trigger points.

- Anywhere you locate tender spots, press the outside muscle fold with a tennis ball or Original Worm, or pinch it between your fingers or the balls of an Acumasseur.

- Hold the pressure for between 10 and 90 seconds per tender spot.

Step 4: Gently Move

Do the movement described on pages 17–18 or the movement below. (See illustrations on opposite page.)

- Stand in a neutral position with the non-treatment side of your body next to a wall. Rest the forearm on the non-treatment side against the wall. The treatment arm is bent at the elbow with the palm facing the body. Take the foot on the treatment side and cross it behind the non-treatment foot; both feet should be flat on the ground. This is your starting position.

- To lengthen the muscle, gently lean your torso away from the wall while bringing your shoulders, head, and treatment arm/palm toward the wall. Your shoulders should remain facing forward. Return to the starting position.

- To shorten the muscle, bring the treatment arm down so that your upper arm is flush against your torso. The elbow should stay bent and the palm should be facing toward you. Return to the starting position.

- Repeat a total of five times.

Other muscles to treat: The serratus anterior (page 122) and sometimes the pectoralis major (page 114), pectoralis minor (page 116), and obliques (page 130).

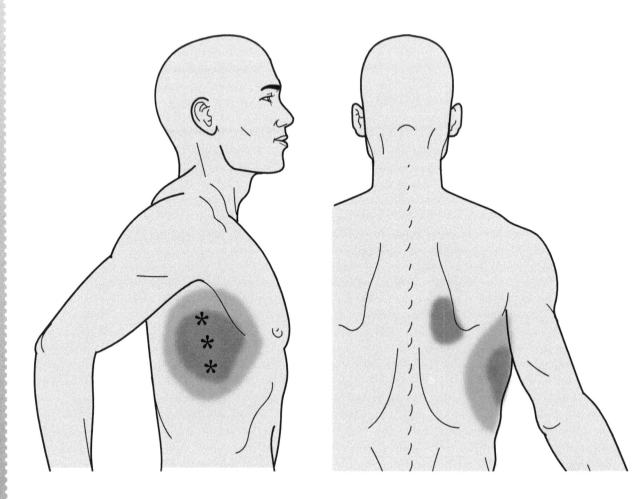

Serratus Anterior

Where it hurts: At the bottom inner edge of your shoulder blade, on the outside portion of your ribs, and down the pinky side of the arm.

You might also be experiencing: Difficulty taking a deep breath, a "stitch in the side" when you run.

It's often caused by: High levels of stress and anxiety, too many push-ups, running long distances, and excessive coughing.

Step 1: **Treat the Spine**

- Using a Big Bend Backnobber, Acumasseur, or Thumbby, apply pressure to the paraspinal muscles in the lower part of your neck, right next to the C5–C7 vertebrae.

Step 2: **Floss the Nerve**

- Floss the long thoracic nerve with the Elbow Bend and Twist nerve floss (page 118).

Step 3: **Treat the Trigger Points**

- Press into the sore spots on the side of the ribs with a tennis ball, racquetball, or Original Worm. (It's also possible to use the Acumasseur here.)

- Hold the pressure for between 10 and 90 seconds per tender spot.

Step 4: **Gently Move**

Do this as a movement without any breaks. (The movement itself will create the breaks.) The directions may seem complicated, but once you start following them, they'll quickly become clear.

- Stand in a neutral position. Gently press your hands and forearms together in front of you with your elbows bent, your fingers pointing up, and your thumbs at nose level. This is your starting position.

- To lengthen the muscle, slowly raise your arms toward the ceiling, keeping them pressed together until they naturally begin to separate.

- Let your arms separate and continue to slowly raise them as high as possible, turning your palms forward at full reach.

- To shorten the muscle, slowly lower your arms, bending your elbows so that they stay pointed downward. Gently squeeze your shoulder blades together as you bring your elbows down.

- Once your elbows are completely lowered, return to the starting position.

- Repeat a total of five times.

Other muscles to treat: Sometimes the pectoralis major (page 114) and pectoralis minor (page 116) can refer pain here.

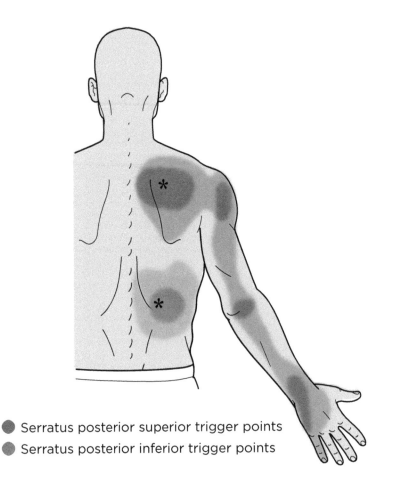

● Serratus posterior superior trigger points
● Serratus posterior inferior trigger points

Serratus Posterior Inferior and Superior

Where it hurts: The lower ribs over the approximate spot where your kidney should be, as well as over the back of your shoulder blade. The pain feels deep.

You might also be experiencing: For the upper muscle (serratus posterior superior), you might have difficulty taking a deep breath or lying on the shoulder blade. For the lower one (serratus posterior inferior), you can often feel a pull when you try to swivel your torso and experience pain when leaning back—say, if you're painting a ceiling.

It's often caused by: Bending and twisting movements.

Step 1: Treat the Spine

- Apply pressure to both the superficial and deep paraspinals between the spine and upper shoulder blade (vertebrae T1–T4) and below the shoulder blade in the rib region (vertebrae T9–T12).

Step 2: Floss the Nerve

- Perform the Slumping for Health nerve floss (page 132).

Step 3: Treat the Trigger Points

- To locate the trigger points, turn your torso and feel for a pull in the lower ribs.

- While seated in a chair with your feet flat on the ground, pull the arm across the chest to expose the superior, which is between the spine and upper shoulder blade. The inferior will be on the lower ribs below the shoulder blade and beside the paraspinals.

- Press with a tennis ball, racquetball, Big Bend Backnobber, or Original Worm. The spots are incredibly tender in these muscles.

- Hold the pressure for between 10 and 90 seconds per tender spot.

Step 4: Gently Move

- Get on all fours and hold your back straight, almost as if you were a table.

- Lengthen the muscle by arching your back with your palms still on the ground. Return to center.

- Shorten the muscle by lifting your head and rounding your belly. Return to center again.

- Repeat a total of five times.

Other muscles to treat: It's sometimes helpful to treat the rhomboids (page 64) and scalenes (page 52).

Tip: The lower muscle (serratus posterior inferior) should not be treated if you have osteoporosis. Talk to your doctor first.

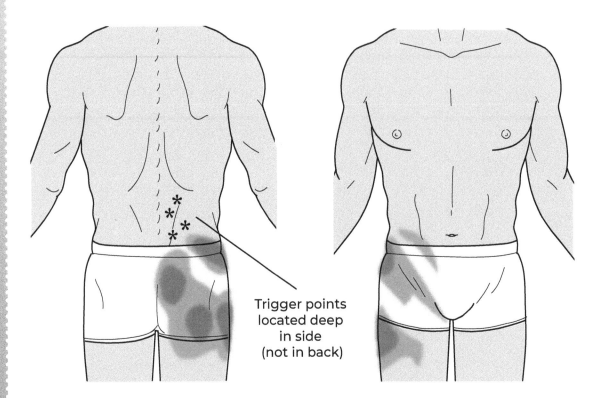

Trigger points located deep in side (not in back)

Quadratus Lumborum

Where it hurts: Over your hip and/or in your buttock.

You might also be experiencing: Difficulty standing up. I've known people who had to crawl on hands and knees to the bathroom because of problems with this muscle.

It's often caused by: Car accidents, falls.

Step 1: **Treat the Spine**

- Using the Big Bend Backnobber or a similar tool, apply pressure to the deep and superficial paraspinal muscles in your lower back, next to the T12–L4 vertebrae.

Step 2: Floss the Nerve

- Perform the Slumping for Health nerve floss (page 132).

Step 3: Treat the Trigger Points

- To find the trigger points, press your fingers straight between your ribs and the top of your pelvis, directly on your side. It will be tender.

- I never use tools for these trigger points. Instead, sit in a chair that has armrests and use them as support for your arms as you apply pressure with your fingers. If you need more pressure, don't press harder; lean away toward the non-treatment side (so if you're working on your right side, lean left).

- Hold the pressure for between 10 and 90 seconds per tender spot.

Step 4: Gently Move

In addition to the movement below, try the nerve floss listed in step 2 of the obliques entry (page 130) as a movement for the deeper fibers of the quadratus lumborum.

- Sit neutrally in a chair with your fingers interlocked in your lap.

- With your palms facing outward and fingers still linked, raise your arms toward the ceiling.

- Lengthen the muscle by pressing one palm upward with fingers still linked. Return to center.

- Shorten the muscle by pressing the other palm upward with fingers still linked. Return to center again.

- Repeat a total of five times.

Other muscles to treat: The iliopsoas (page 140) and sometimes the tensor fasciae latae (page 136) or rectus femoris (page 138).

Tip: It is extremely important to use only your fingers on this muscle. Using a massage tool here can break a rib!

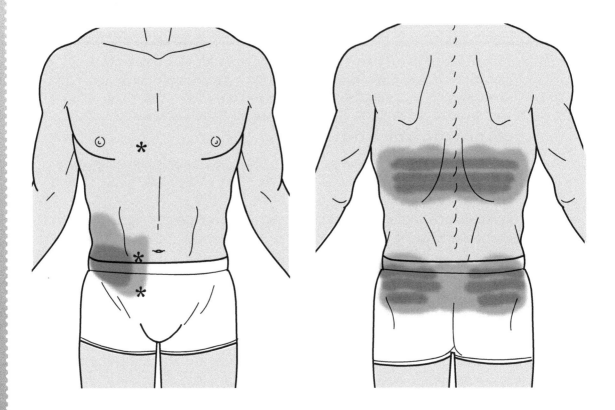

Rectus Abdominis

Where it hurts: Across the lower ribs and back.

You might also be experiencing: Nausea, vomiting, heartburn, and cramping.

It's often caused by: Stress, internal issues (peptic ulcers, tapeworm), and physical trauma (this doesn't mean only slips or falls—even lifesaving surgery can be a trauma).

Step 1: Treat the Spine

- Using the Big Bend Backnobber or a similar tool, apply pressure to the paraspinal muscles in the rib region below the shoulder blade (vertebrae T7–T12).

Step 2: Floss the Nerve

- Get on all fours with your back straight, almost as if you were a table. (If you can't get on all fours, modify by putting your arms on a table instead.)

- With your palms still flat on the ground, gently arch your back up, kind of like a scared cat. Return to neutral.

- Then do the opposite: Slowly round your belly down toward the floor while gently lifting your head. Return to neutral again.

- Repeat a total of 10 times.

Step 3: Treat the Trigger Points

- Stand in a neutral position, then put your hands on your hips and lean slightly backward. You should be able to feel where this muscle is tight.

- Press your fingers in a line where you feel the tightness in your stomach. Taking a deep breath into your belly and holding it makes it easier to find the tender spots.

- Hold the pressure for between 10 and 90 seconds per tender spot.

Step 4: Gently Move

- Perform the nerve floss in step 2 a total of five times.

Other muscles to treat: The obliques (page 130) and sometimes the tensor fasciae latae (page 136) or rectus femoris (page 138).

Tip: Consult with a doctor if you're having stomach pains, especially if you're experiencing internal problems like diarrhea, vomiting, or dysmenorrhea. Trigger points might be involved, but you might also have serious internal issues like ulcers or appendicitis that require medical treatment.

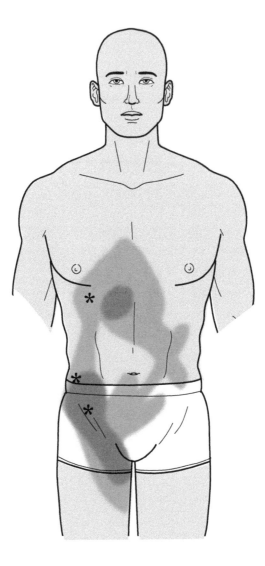

Obliques

Where it hurts: Anywhere in the abdomen, all the way down to the groin/testicular region.

You might also be experiencing: Heartburn, belching.

It's often caused by: Emotional stress, abdominal diseases like ulcers or appendicitis, physical trauma.

Step 1: Treat the Spine

- Using the Big Bend Backnobber or a similar tool, apply pressure to the paraspinal muscles in the rib region below the shoulder blade (vertebrae T8–T12).

Step 2: Floss the Nerve

- Start by sitting in a neutral position.

- Exhale as you slowly and gently turn your torso to the left. Return to neutral.

- Exhale as you slowly and gently turn your torso to the right. Return to neutral again.

- Repeat a total of 10 times.

Step 3: Treat the Trigger Points

- Press into any tender spots on your lower ribs with a tennis ball or Thumbby.

- Hold the pressure for between 10 and 90 seconds per tender spot.

Step 4: Gently Move

- Perform the nerve floss in step 2 a total of five times.

Other muscles to treat: The rectus abdominis (page 128), iliopsoas (page 140), and occasionally the tensor fasciae latae (page 136) or rectus femoris (page 138).

Tip: Consult with a doctor if you're having stomach pains, especially if you're experiencing internal problems like diarrhea, vomiting, or dysmenorrhea. Trigger points might be involved, but you might also have serious internal issues like ulcers or appendicitis.

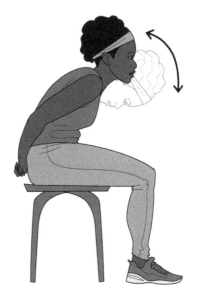

NERVE FLOSS: Slumping for Health

This movement flosses the segmental nerves in your spine that supply your paraspinal muscles (pages 110 and 112)— those muscles all along the sides of your spine that you massage in step 1 of almost every entry in this book. Because your nerves connect all your muscles to your brain through your spine, this nerve floss benefits not just your paraspinals but also your entire body.

Instructions

- Sit in a slumped position with your shoulders rounded forward and your head hanging. Join your hands behind your back, using one hand (it doesn't matter which) to gently grasp the opposite wrist.

- Maintaining your slumped position, inhale as you gently tilt your head upward and look at the ceiling.

- Exhale as you gently lower your head back down to the starting position. Wherever you feel a pull, that's where the nerve is not moving with the muscles the way it should be.

- Repeat a total of 10 times.

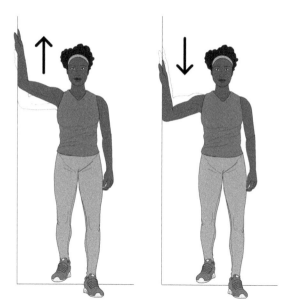

NERVE FLOSS: Doorway Step

This movement flosses the medial and lateral pectoral nerves in your shoulder that supply the pectoralis major (page 114) and minor (page 116).

Instructions

- Stand in a doorway or next to a wall with your treatment side next to the doorframe or wall. Your treatment-side foot should be slightly behind you, with the other foot slightly in front of you. Raise your treatment arm, bend your elbow at a 90-degree angle, and place your forearm against the wall or doorframe. Make sure your elbow stays level with your shoulder.

- Bend the knee of the leg in front until you feel a mild pull in your pectoral muscles as you gently bring your ear toward your shoulder on the treatment side. Then return to the starting position.

- Move your forearm slightly up the wall so that your elbow is above your shoulder and repeat the gentle movement.

- Now move your forearm slightly down the wall so that your elbow is below your shoulder.

- Repeat a total of 10 times. Though it is only essential to do this floss on the treatment side, it is best if done on both sides.

CHAPTER SEVEN

Hips and Upper Legs

A lot of things can contribute to trigger point pain in your hips and upper legs, including athletic injuries, falls, sacroiliac dysfunction (problems with your hip joints), and lower back conditions such as issues with the discs or joints in your spine. Self-treatment is essential to full recovery in many of these conditions, and this chapter will show you how to do just that.

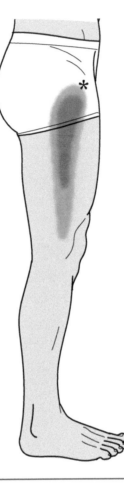

Tensor Fasciae Latae (TFL)

Where it hurts: Your hip and the outside of your thigh.

You might also be experiencing: Difficulty sleeping on your side, lower back pain, and numbness on the outside of your thigh.

It's often caused by: Sleeping in the fetal position or sitting with your knees above your hips, as you might if you're a tall person with a low office chair or a teacher who frequently sits in children's chairs. I had an older couple whose back pain stopped after they replaced a really low couch.

Step 1: **Treat the Spine**

- Using a Big Bend Backnobber, Original Worm, or tennis ball, apply pressure to the paraspinal muscles in the lower back, right next to vertebrae L4–S1.

Step 2: **Floss the Nerve**

- Floss the femoral nerve with the Heel to Butt nerve floss (page 157).

Step 3: **Treat the Trigger Points**

- Find the hip bone that juts out in front on the treatment side—it's called the anterior superior iliac spine, or ASIS. You should be able to find tender spots an inch or two to the outside and just below this bone.

- Trap a tennis ball or the Original Worm between the muscle and a doorframe or wall. Angle the other side of your body away so that your face isn't against the wall.

- Hold the pressure for between 10 and 90 seconds per tender spot.

Step 4: **Gently Move**

- Stand in a neutral position by a wall so you can use it for balance.

- To lengthen the muscle, gently turn your torso away from the treatment side, keeping your legs in place.

- Return to neutral.

- To shorten the muscle, gently turn your torso toward the treatment side, keeping your legs in place.

- Return to neutral again.

- Repeat a total of five times.

Other muscles to treat: Sometimes the iliopsoas (page 140) or rectus femoris (page 138) can refer pain here.

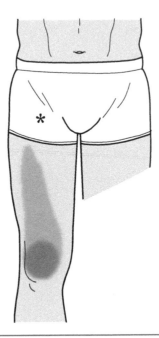

Rectus Femoris

Where it hurts: The front of the knee.

You might also be experiencing: Lower back pain, weakness going downstairs.

It's often caused by: Falls, skiing accidents.

Step 1: **Treat the Spine**

- Using the Big Bend Backnobber or a similar tool, apply pressure to the paraspinal muscles in the lower back, right next to vertebrae L2–L4.

Step 2: **Floss the Nerve**

- Use the Heel to Butt nerve floss (page 157) to floss the femoral nerve.

Step 3: **Treat the Trigger Points**

- You can feel the tight region when you gently pull your heel toward your buttock while standing.

- Find the hip bone that juts out in front on the treatment side—it's called the anterior superior iliac spine, or ASIS. You should be able to find tender spots an inch or two below that in the center of your thigh.

- Use a tennis ball or Original Worm to apply pressure for 10 to 90 seconds per tender spot.

Step 4: Gently Move

Try the movement in step 4 of the gluteus maximus entry (page 146), or use the one below.

- Start by lying on a bed with the treatment leg close to the edge. (See illustrations below.)

- To lengthen the muscle, let the treatment leg gently hang over the edge of the bed. Return to neutral.

- To shorten the muscle, bend the knee of the treatment leg and use your hands to gently pull it up toward the opposite shoulder. Return to neutral.

- Repeat a total of five times.

Other muscles to treat: Sometimes it can be helpful to treat the tensor fasciae latae (page 136), vastus muscles (page 142), or iliopsoas (page 140).

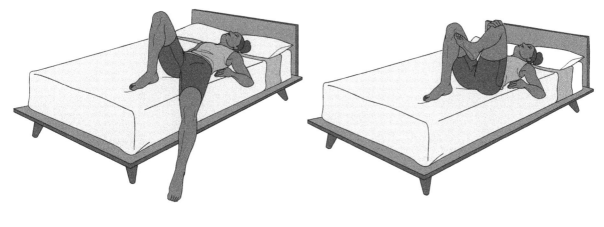

Lengthen   Shorten

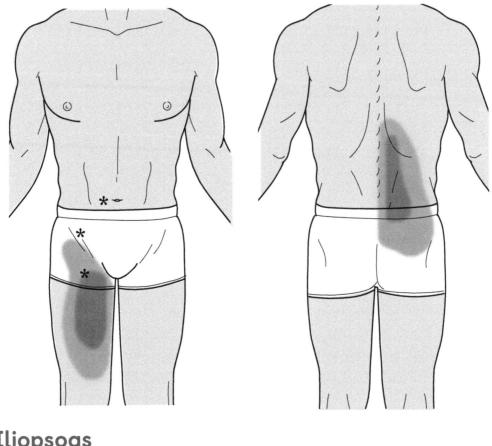

Iliopsoas
Iliacus, Psoas

Where it hurts: In the lower spine and/or upper front of the thigh.

You might also be experiencing: Tingling on the outside of your thigh, difficulty getting out of a chair, inability to stand straight at the waist.

It's often caused by: Stress or physical strain on the hips, especially during exercise. I once had a patient with severe lower back pain whose physical therapist started him with sit-ups. The patient thought that if 30 sit-ups were good for him, 750 would be exceptional. I treated him *and* limited the sit-ups to 50 a day—that did the trick!

Step 1: **Treat the Spine**

- Using the Big Bend Backnobber or a similar tool, apply pressure to the paraspinal muscles in the lower back, right next to vertebrae L2–L4.

Step 2: Floss the Nerve

- Floss the femoral nerve with the Heel to Butt nerve floss (page 157).

Step 3: Treat the Trigger Points

- To check where your trigger points are, sit on a bed, hang the treatment leg over the side of the bed, and pull the opposite knee to the chest. If the treatment leg hangs against the bed, it should be fine. If it's in the air, the muscle is too tight.

- Once you've located your tender spots, stand in a doorframe and put a medium-size ball between your belly button and the bone that juts out in front of your hip on the treatment side. The ball should be bigger than a tennis ball but smaller than a volleyball (I get mine from the toy store).

- Step your non-treatment foot through the doorway, like you're doing a gentle lunge stretch. The ball should be pressed in between your body and the doorframe, applying pressure to any tender spots.

- Hold the pressure for between 10 and 90 seconds per tender spot.

Step 4: Gently Move

- For the psoas (inner) portion of the muscle, stand in a "fencer" position with the treatment leg back and the other leg forward. For the iliacus (outer) portion, do the same position but turn the back leg so the foot faces inward (you may need to hold on to something for balance).

- Lengthen the muscle by gently bending the front leg and tipping the front of the pelvis toward the sky until you feel a slight pull. Return to neutral.

- Shorten the muscle by gently bending your torso forward at the hips.

- Return to neutral.

Other muscles to treat: The tensor fasciae latae (page 136), the rectus femoris (page 138), and occasionally the quadratus lumborum (page 126).

Tip: This is a stubborn one. I'd also do one of the breathing exercises on page 22.

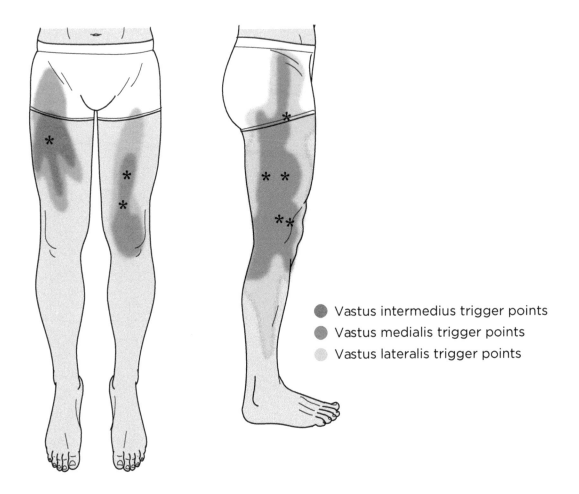

● Vastus intermedius trigger points
● Vastus medialis trigger points
● Vastus lateralis trigger points

Vastus Muscles
Vastus Medialis, Vastus Lateralis, Vastus Intermedius

Where it hurts: On both the inner and outer sides of the knee and thigh.

You might also be experiencing: Buckling knees (from trigger points on the inner side of the knee) and/or locking of the knees (from trigger points on the outer side).

It's often caused by: Getting tackled, falling, being kicked in the knee.

Step 1: **Treat the Spine**

- Using the Big Bend Backnobber or a similar tool, apply pressure to the paraspinal muscles in the lower back, right next to vertebrae L2–L4.

Step 2: **Floss the Nerve**

- Floss the femoral nerve with the Heel to Butt nerve floss (page 157).

Step 3: **Treat the Trigger Points**

- Start by lying on your back and bringing your heel toward your butt. If these muscles are healthy, you should be able to touch your butt with your heel. If you can't, notice where you feel tightness.

- Search the tight area for trigger points. You should find them on the inside of the front of the knee and/or on the outer side of the entire thigh.

- I like to use the Tiger Tail or Acumasseur to apply pressure here, but you can also use your elbow (for the inside of your knee) or lie on your side on a tennis ball (for the outside of your thigh).

- Hold the pressure for between 10 and 90 seconds per tender spot.

Step 4: **Gently Move**

See page 139 in the rectus femoris entry for illustrations.

- Start by lying on a bed with the treatment leg close to the edge.

- To lengthen the muscle, let the treatment leg gently hang over the edge of the bed. Return to neutral.

- To shorten the muscle, bend the knee of the treatment leg and use your hands to gently pull it up toward the opposite shoulder. Return to neutral.

- Repeat a total of five times.

Other muscles to treat: Sometimes it helps to treat the rectus femoris (page 138) or the outside hamstring (page 154).

Tip: If one of your thighs is smaller than the other, you might have a number of issues unrelated to trigger points. You'll want to visit an orthopedic doctor. (If you're not sure about the size of your thighs, you can measure your thigh with a cloth measuring tape. Take measurements at 4 and 6 inches above the middle of the kneecap, then compare sides.)

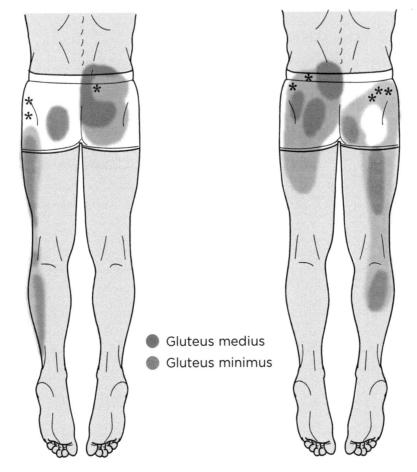

● Gluteus medius
● Gluteus minimus

Gluteus Medius and Minimus

Where it hurts: In the buttock and down the back and/or side of the leg.

You might also be experiencing: If you sit on the floor with your legs in front of you, you might not be able to roll the inside of the foot to the floor. Your feet could also turn out, like a duck's. It can be hard to sleep on your side because of tossing and turning from the pain.

It's often caused by: Falls, sports injuries, nerve irritation, and sacroiliac joint dysfunction (issues with your hip joints).

Step 1: **Treat the Spine**

- Using the Big Bend Backnobber or a similar tool, apply pressure to the paraspinal muscles in the lower back, right next to vertebrae L4–S1.

Step 2: **Floss the Nerve**

- Perform the Lean and Look nerve floss (page 158) to floss the sciatic nerve.

Step 3: **Treat the Trigger Points**

- Lie on the floor on your back with the treatment leg straight and the other knee bent. Your tennis ball or Original Worm goes under the bone at the top of your butt/pelvis, between your tailbone and hip bone.

- Keep moving the ball to feel for tender spots. Hold the pressure for between 10 and 90 seconds per tender spot.

- If you need more pressure, press the other foot down. You can also roll over onto your side and press between the hip bone and the bone at the bottom of your waist. That area has more effect on the outside of the leg.

Step 4: **Gently Move**

- Start on your hands and knees with your hands shoulder-width apart and your knees hip-width apart, looking down at the floor.

- To lengthen the muscle, straighten the treatment leg and bring it slightly out to the side with the toe still touching the ground. Return to center.

- To shorten the muscle, straighten the treatment leg and cross it slightly over the non-treatment leg, resting the toe on the ground. Return to center.

- Repeat a total of five times.

Other muscles to treat: Sometimes the quadratus lumborum (page 126) can refer pain here.

Tip: If you feel numbness or tingling, it means you've rolled the ball onto a nerve. Move the ball slightly and try again.

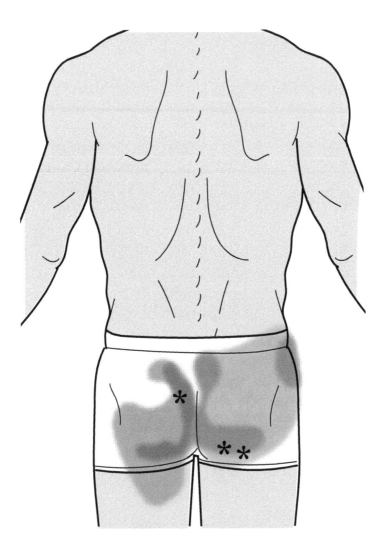

Gluteus Maximus

Where it hurts: In your buttocks.

You might also be experiencing: Trigger points in this area limit your ability to bring your knee toward your opposite shoulder while you're lying on your back. If it's really bad, you might have difficulty bending over to tie your shoes or crossing the treatment leg over the other. Sometimes these trigger points team up with your hamstrings to create a flat back.

It's often caused by: Falling on your bum!

Step 1: Treat the Spine

- Using the Big Bend Backnobber or a similar tool, apply pressure to the deep paraspinal muscles in the lower back, right next to vertebrae L5–S2.

Step 2: Floss the Nerve

- Perform the Sitting Toe Pointer nerve floss (page 159).

Step 3: Treat the Trigger Points

- Apply pressure to any tender spots on the treatment side just above the bones you sit on (otherwise known as the ischial tuberosity or "sit bones"). You can do this with a tennis ball or the Original Worm while leaning against a wall or lying on your back.

- Hold the pressure for between 10 and 90 seconds per tender spot.

Step 4: Gently Move

Use the movement in step 4 of the iliopsoas entry or the one below.

- Lie on your non-treatment side on a flat surface.

- Lengthen the muscle by gently bringing your treatment knee toward your chest. Return to center.

- Shorten the muscle by gently extending your treatment leg straight behind you. Return to center again.

- Repeat a total of five times.

Other muscles to treat: The quadratus lumborum (page 126) and sometimes the iliopsoas (page 140) or tensor fasciae latae (page 136).

Tip: If you experience numbness or tingling in the leg while doing this, you're probably pressing the ball onto a nerve. Move the ball slightly and try again.

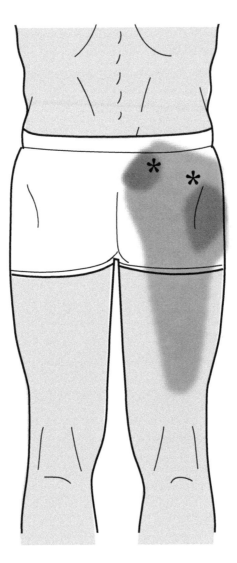

Piriformis

Where it hurts: In the buttocks, over the hip, and down the back of the thigh.

You might also be experiencing: Numbness and tingling in the leg, in addition to pain when pressing the gas pedal, making love, or sleeping on your side. If you sit on the floor with your legs straight out in front, the tightness often prevents you from turning the inside of your foot toward the ground.

It's often caused by: Car accidents, falls, constant shortening of the muscle when driving.

Step 1: **Treat the Spine**

- Using the Big Bend Backnobber or a similar tool, apply pressure to the deep paraspinal muscles in the very lowest part of the back, right next to vertebrae S1–S2.

Step 2: **Floss the Nerve**

- Do either the Lean and Look nerve floss (page 158) or the Sitting Toe Pointer nerve floss (page 159)—whichever one seems to work better for you.

Step 3: **Treat the Trigger Points**

- While leaning against the wall or lying flat on the floor, put a tennis ball or Original Worm between you and the surface. Use it to press any tender spots just above and a little inward from the top of the hip bone (on the side or in the back).

- Hold the pressure for between 10 and 90 seconds per tender spot.

Step 4: **Gently Move**

- Sit in a neutral position on the edge of a chair.

- Lengthen the muscle by crossing the treatment-side knee over the other knee. Return to neutral.

- Shorten the muscle by gently bringing the knee out to the side, sliding the foot along the floor. Return to neutral again.

- Repeat a total of five times.

Other muscles to treat: The gluteus maximus (page 146), gluteus medius and minimus (page 144), or quadratus lumborum (page 126).

Tip: If you feel numbness and tingling while trying to treat this muscle, talk to a professional.

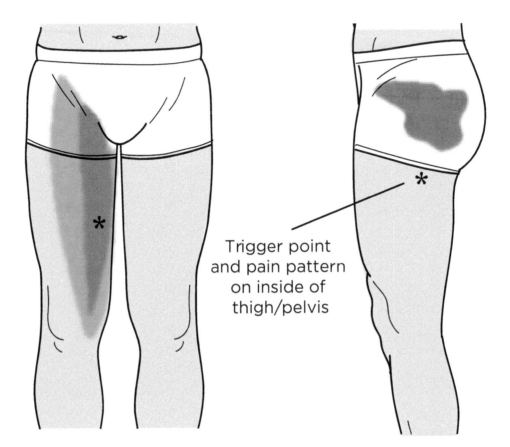

Trigger point
and pain pattern
on inside of
thigh/pelvis

Adductor Magnus

Where it hurts: The inside of the thigh, sometimes inside the pelvis.

You might also be experiencing: The inability to touch your toes, hamstrings that never seem to release. Often, making love is not possible when the legs can't separate far enough.

It's often caused by: Stress—you instinctively curl up in a ball to protect yourself. People rarely use this muscle through its full motion, so it shortens to accommodate what you usually do.

Step 1: Treat the Spine

- Using the Big Bend Backnobber or a similar tool, apply pressure to the paraspinal muscles in the lower back, right next to vertebrae L4–S1.

Step 2: Floss the Nerve

- To floss the obturator nerve, start by sitting in a neutral position on the edge of a chair with your knees bent.

- Exhale as you slowly raise the treatment knee, bringing it out to the treatment side as you go. At the same time, slowly look up and twist your torso to the non-treatment side. Return to neutral.

- Repeat a total of 10 times.

Step 3: Treat the Trigger Points

- To find the trigger points, sit on the edge of a chair with your feet on the ground. Place your hand on the treatment knee and gently twist away from it. While twisting, you should be able to feel where it's tight.

- Lie on your non-treatment side. Place a tennis ball or Original Worm on a small step stool or pile of books—whatever will bring it to the height of your thigh. Line the ball up with your trigger point.

- Bring your thigh forward and rest it on the ball. The weight of your thigh is all the pressure you need. (Remember not to apply pressure directly on a pulse.)

- Hold the pressure for between 10 and 90 seconds per tender spot.

Step 4: Gently Move

- Start by sitting neutrally on the edge of a chair with your knees bent.

- Exhale as you slowly raise the treatment knee, bringing it out to the treatment side as you go. Return to neutral.

- Exhale as you slowly straighten the treatment knee and cross your foot over to the non-treatment side. Return to neutral.

- Repeat a total of five times.

Other muscles to treat: The adductor longus (page 152).

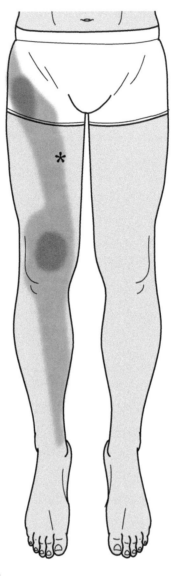

Adductor Longus

Where it hurts: The inside of the thigh, leg, and groin.

You might also be experiencing: Difficulty with activities that involve moving your knees outward, such as riding a horse or sitting cross-legged.

It's often caused by: Physical trauma like falling on ice; spending a long time sitting, especially with the legs crossed.

Step 1: Treat the Spine

- Using the Big Bend Backnobber or a similar tool, apply pressure to the paraspinal muscles in the lower back, right next to vertebrae L2–L4.

Step 2: Floss the Nerve

- To floss the obturator nerve, start by sitting in a neutral position on the edge of a chair with your knees bent.

- Exhale as you slowly raise the treatment knee, bringing it out to the treatment side as you go. Slowly look up and twist your torso to the non-treatment side as you move. Return to neutral.

- Repeat a total of 10 times.

Step 3: Treat the Trigger Points

- Lie on your non-treatment side. Place a tennis ball or Original Worm on a small step stool or pile of books—whatever will bring it to the height of your thigh. Line the ball up with your trigger point.

- Bring your thigh forward and rest it on the ball. The weight of your thigh is all the pressure you need.

- Hold the pressure for between 10 and 90 seconds per tender spot.

Step 4: Gently Move

- Start by sitting in a neutral position on the edge of a chair with your knees bent.

- Exhale as you slowly raise the treatment knee, bringing it out to the treatment side as you go. Return to neutral.

- Exhale as you slowly straighten the treatment knee and cross your foot over to the non-treatment side. Return to neutral.

- Repeat a total of five times.

Other muscles to treat: The adductor magnus (page 150).

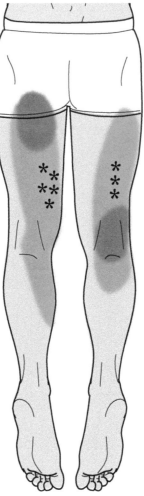

Hamstrings
Biceps Femoris, Semitendinosus, Semimembranosus

Where it hurts: The back of your upper thigh and the lower buttock (from trigger points on the inside fibers); the back of the knee (from trigger points in the fibers of the outer edge).

You might also be experiencing: Knee pain, if the outside hamstring has twisted the knee out of alignment.

It's often caused by: Tightness in the rectus and vastus muscles.

Step 1: Treat the Spine

- Using the Big Bend Backnobber or a similar tool, apply pressure to the paraspinal muscles in the very lowest part of the back, right next to vertebrae L5–S2.

Step 2: Floss the Nerve

- Do either the Lean and Look nerve floss (page 158) or the Sitting Toe Pointer nerve floss (page 159)—whichever seems to work better for you.

Step 3: Treat the Trigger Points

- To find the trigger points, start by standing in a neutral position. Put the treatment leg in front of you and gently lean toward your toes, feeling for where it's tight.

- Then angle the leg inward and repeat to test the outer fibers of the hamstring. Repeat one more time with your leg angled outward to test the inside fibers.

- Before you treat the trigger points, put your leg out straight while sitting. Make one mark in the center of your kneecap and another on your shinbone just below the knee. If the lower mark is on the outer side of the leg, treat only the hamstring muscles on the outer side of your leg.

- Feel for tender spots in the area(s) where you felt tightness, then apply pressure and/or squeeze. I love to trap the fibers with the Acumasseur. You can also put a tennis ball or Original Worm under your thigh and sit on a hard chair.

- Hold the pressure for between 10 and 90 seconds per tender spot.

Step 4: Gently Move

- Sit neutrally in a chair with the treatment leg extended in front of you, heel on the ground. (See illustrations on next page.)

- To lengthen the muscle, keep it straight, but slide the heel to the outside (if the inner fibers of the hamstring are tight) or to the inside (if the outer fibers of the hamstring are tight). Return to neutral.

Continued

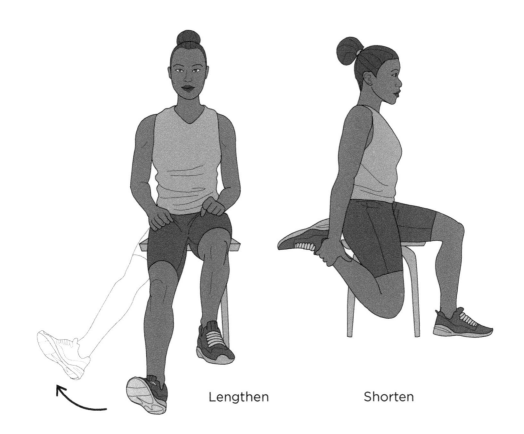

Lengthen   Shorten

- To shorten the muscle, turn your entire body to the non-treatment side so you're sitting sideways in the chair. Keep the non-treatment leg in a neutral position in front of you with the knee bent and the foot flat on the ground. Use your hand to gently pull the ankle of the treatment leg toward the buttock so that the knee of the treatment leg is hanging over the front of the chair.

- Repeat a total of five times.

Other muscles to treat: The adductor magnus (page 150), rectus femoris (page 138), and vastus muscles (page 142).

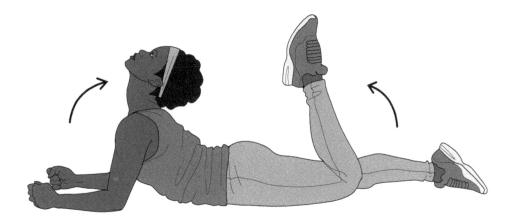

NERVE FLOSS: Heel to Butt

This movement flosses your femoral nerve, which supplies muscles in your abdomen and anterior thigh, such as the iliopsoas (page 140), rectus femoris (page 138), and vastus muscles (page 142). The flossing movement calms the nerve that controls those muscles and is helpful for pain in the lower back, thigh, and knee.

Instructions

- Lie on your stomach with your forearms on the ground.

- Exhale as you use your arms to slowly lift the front half of your body, keeping your hips on the ground.

- At the same time, gently tilt your face toward the ceiling and slowly bring the heel on the treatment side toward the buttock.

- Repeat a total of 10 times.

Tip: If you find it hard to get up off the floor, you might want to do this nerve floss on your bed.

NERVE FLOSS: Lean and Look

This movement flosses the sciatic nerve in your leg that supplies a number of muscles in the foot, calf, posterior thigh, and buttock.

Instructions

- Stand facing a wall with your feet shoulder-width apart, your arms at your sides, and your shoulders relaxed, gazing straight ahead. Your toes should be about six inches from the wall.

- Take the treatment-side foot and place it so that the ball of the foot is against the wall with the heel of the foot on the ground.

- Slowly lean your body slightly forward. As you lean, also look up, raising your chin slightly.

- Exhale as you move forward. Repeat 10 times.

Tip: You can change this up a bit by changing the position of your foot. Angling your foot a bit to the left or right at the beginning of the floss can change the angle of pull on the nerve. You can feel it in the back of the calf and, with practice, in the buttock.

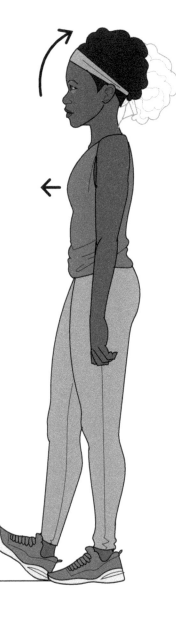

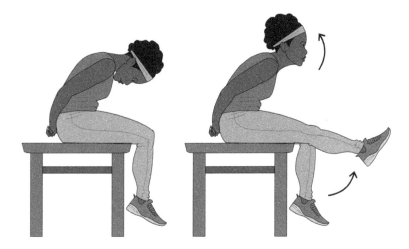

NERVE FLOSS: Sitting Toe Pointer

This movement flosses the spinal, tibial, and peroneal nerves, and is particularly helpful for pain in the gluteus maximus (page 146), paraspinals (pages 110 and 112), hamstrings (page 154), and everything below the knee (see chapter 8).

Instructions

- Start by sitting on the edge of a bed or in a chair high enough so your feet dangle rather than fully touching the floor. Sit in a gently slumped position with your hands gently clasped behind your back.

- Without straightening your back, exhale as you slowly tilt your head back and look up.

- At the same time, slowly straighten the knee on the treatment side and lift your foot off the ground. If your problem is in the peroneals, ankle/toe extensors, and/or dorsal foot muscles, point your toes during this. If your problem is in the gastrocnemius, soleus, tibialis posterior, ankle/toe flexors, and/or plantar foot muscles, you'll want your foot gently flexed. Some people require both motions. It doesn't matter how high off the ground your foot goes, so don't strain yourself.

- Repeat a total of 10 times.

CHAPTER EIGHT

Lower Legs and Feet

Are you dealing with hammertoes, shin splints, or plantar fasciitis? Do you wear high heels, wake up in the middle of the night with pain in your calf, or just really need a good foot rub? If you answered yes to any of those questions, you're in the right place. Trigger points are often associated with pain in the feet, ankles, and lower legs. Be sure to look at the pictures carefully to find just the right place to press!

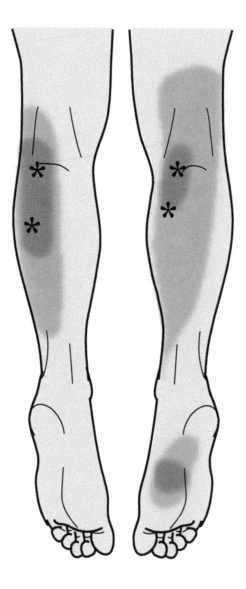

Gastrocnemius

Where it hurts: The upper calf, back of the knee, and bottom of the instep of the foot.

You might also be experiencing: Calf cramps that wake you up at night.

It's often caused by: Wearing high heels, sitting with your feet dangling.

Step 1: **Treat the Spine**

• Using the Big Bend Backnobber or a similar tool, apply pressure to the paraspinal muscles in the deep lower back, right next to vertebrae S1–S2.

Step 2: **Floss the Nerve**

• Do the Sitting Toe Pointer nerve floss (page 159) and/or the Lean and Look nerve floss (page 158).

Step 3: **Treat the Trigger Points**

• At the top of the calf on either side, rub across the muscle from side to side to locate the tender region.

• Apply pressure. This is a great place to gently squeeze the inner side and outer side separately with the Acumasseur. You can also straighten your leg in front of you and place a tennis ball or Original Worm under the calf. If you need more pressure, cross your ankles.

• Hold the pressure for between 10 and 90 seconds per tender spot.

Step 4: **Gently Move**

• Do the Lean and Look nerve floss (page 158) a total of five times.

Other muscles to treat: Sometimes it helps to treat the gluteus minimus (page 144) or soleus (page 164).

Tips

• Avoid pointing your toes when you stretch before getting out of bed. You can bring them toward your knees instead.

• Many people find that putting pillows under the covers at the foot of the bed makes a tent so that the weight of the covers doesn't cause the toes to point.

• If this muscle is red, warm, or swollen, don't press it! See your doctor as soon as possible.

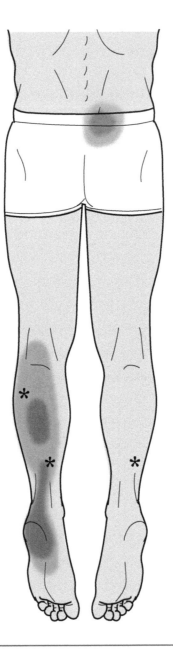

Soleus

Where it hurts: Your calf and heel.

You might also be experiencing: Pain when you put weight on your heel or when using stairs.

It's often caused by: Wearing high heels, sitting with your feet dangling.

Step 1: **Treat the Spine**

- Using the Big Bend Backnobber or a similar tool, apply pressure to the paraspinal muscles in the deep lower back, right next to vertebrae S1–S2.

Step 2: **Floss the Nerve**

- Do the Sitting Toe Pointer nerve floss (page 159) and/or the Lean and Look nerve floss (page 158).

Step 3: **Treat the Trigger Points**

- Sit in a chair and slide your finger up from your Achilles tendon (the thick tendon in the back of your heel) to where it begins to split (about a hand's width above the top of the heel). Move your finger one finger's width up and one finger's width toward the outside of the leg. Then do the same on the opposite side, but go up two fingers' width from the spot where the Achilles tendon starts to split.

- Apply pressure at the tender spot. You can straighten your leg on the ground in front of you and place a tennis ball or Original Worm under the calf. If you need more pressure, cross your ankles.

- Hold the pressure for between 10 and 90 seconds per tender spot.

Step 4: **Gently Move**

- Sit in a chair in a neutral position with your feet shoulder-width apart.

- To lengthen the muscle, exhale as you slowly bend the treatment ankle, flexing the toes so that they point up toward your nose. Return to neutral.

- To shorten the muscle, exhale as you slowly extend the treatment ankle, this time pointing your toes forward toward the floor. Return to neutral again.

- Repeat a total of five times.

Other muscles to treat: Sometimes the gluteus minimus (page 144) can refer pain here.

Tip: If your calf is red, warm, or swollen, don't press it! You need to see your doctor.

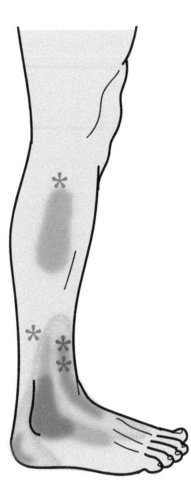

Peroneus Muscles

Where it hurts: Around the outer side of the anklebone and sometimes the instep where the ankle and foot meet.

You might also be experiencing: Frequent ankle sprains. You can often feel the tightness when you put your foot in a neutral position (as when standing) and turn your ankle toward the other foot.

It's often caused by: A history of ankle sprains, and equestrian injury— the instep pain often happens when a horse steps there.

Step 1: Treat the Spine

- Using the Big Bend Backnobber or a similar tool, apply pressure to the paraspinal muscles in the deep lower back, right next to vertebrae L4–S1.

Step 2: Floss the Nerve

- Do the Sitting Toe Pointer nerve floss (page 159) and/or the Lean and Look nerve floss (page 158).

Step 3: Treat the Trigger Points

- There are three regions where you can press: (1) on the outer side of your leg, about three fingers' width below the bony protuberance just below the side of your knee; (2) a hand's width above the ankle on the side of the leg; or (3) a hand's width above the ankle on the front of the leg. Treat whichever one is tender.

- When you've selected your area(s), apply pressure. I like to roll over the side of the leg with a Tiger Tail or lie on my side with a racquetball or tennis ball on the spot.

- Hold the pressure for between 10 and 90 seconds.

Step 4: Gently Move

- Sit in a chair or on a bed in a neutral position.

- To lengthen the muscle, exhale as you slowly straighten your treatment leg in front of you, turning the insole of the treatment foot toward the non-treatment side. Return to neutral.

- To shorten the muscle, exhale as you keep your heel in place, but slowly move the toes of the treatment foot outward, away from the midline. Return to neutral again.

- Repeat a total of five times.

Other muscles to treat: The gluteus minimus (page 144).

Tip: Don't apply pressure to the upper third of the outer side of your leg below your knee. The nerve that controls your ability to lift your toes goes through this area. I once saw a patient who used a rolling pin over the nerve and developed a foot drop.

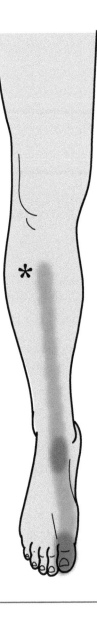

Tibialis Anterior

Where it hurts: Both the instep and the big toe (a condition sometimes called "turf toe").

You might also be experiencing: Weak ankles, foot drop, and/or scuffing on the top of your shoes from dragging your foot. It's sometimes mistaken for compartment syndrome or shin splints.

It's often caused by: An ankle sprain, tripping.

Step 1: Treat the Spine

- Using the Big Bend Backnobber or a similar tool, apply pressure to the paraspinal muscles in the deep lower back, right next to vertebrae L4–S1.

Step 2: Floss the Nerve

- Perform the Sitting Toe Pointer nerve floss (page 159).

Step 3: Treat the Trigger Points

- If you put your leg straight in front of you and point your toes, you'll feel the pull that indicates the trigger point just on the outside of the shin.

- Press the tender area where you feel the pull with a finger or Thumbby. The Tiger Tail can be rolled over this region as well.

- Hold the pressure for between 10 and 90 seconds per tender spot.

Step 4: Gently Move

- Sit in a chair in a neutral position with your treatment leg out in front of you, knee straight or slightly bent, heel resting on the floor.

- To lengthen the muscle, exhale as you slowly extend the treatment ankle, keeping your heel in place as you point your toes forward toward the floor. Then let the ankle relax.

- To shorten the muscle, exhale as you slowly flex the foot on the treatment side so that your toes point up toward your nose. Then let the ankle relax again.

- Repeat a total of five times.

Other muscles to treat: The gluteus minimus (page 144).

Tip: Pain in the leg may indicate a deeper problem, like compartment syndrome. Consult with a doctor to determine the cause of your pain.

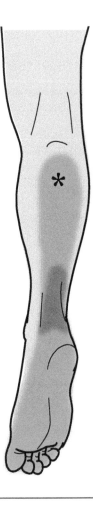

Tibialis Posterior

Where it hurts: The Achilles tendon (the thick tendon in the back of your heel) and sometimes the bottom of the foot.

You might also be experiencing: Inability to stand on tiptoe, as you might while reaching for a high shelf. You might fail to "toe walk" during a test at the doctor's office. Some people's feet have high arches that disappear when they stand up.

It's often caused by: Wearing old shoes that don't support your feet; running on uneven surfaces, like trails or the beach.

Step 1: Treat the Spine

- Using the Big Bend Backnobber or a similar tool, apply pressure to the paraspinal muscles in the deep lower back, right next to vertebrae L5–S1.

Step 2: Floss the Nerve

- Do the Sitting Toe Pointer nerve floss (page 159) and/or the Lean and Look nerve floss (page 158).

Step 3: Treat the Trigger Points

- To find your trigger point, place a belt around the bottom of your foot. Without pointing your toes, pull the outer side of your foot outward, away from your midline. If it doesn't move, the muscle is tight—but you might not feel it.

- Cross the ankle on the treatment side over the opposite knee. The tender region is just behind the tibia, or shinbone.

- Press between the bone and the overlying gastrocnemius (page 162) and soleus (page 164) muscles with either your thumbs or the Thumbby.

- Hold the pressure for between 10 and 90 seconds per tender spot.

Step 4: Gently Move

- Sit in a chair in a neutral position with your treatment leg out in front of you, knee straight or slightly bent, heel resting on the floor.

- To lengthen the muscle, exhale as you slowly flex the treatment ankle so that your toes point up toward your nose. Then let the ankle relax.

- To shorten the muscle, exhale as you slowly extend the treatment ankle, pointing your toes forward toward the floor. Then let the ankle relax again.

- Repeat a total of five times.

Other muscles to treat: The gastrocnemius (page 162) or soleus (page 164) can refer pain here.

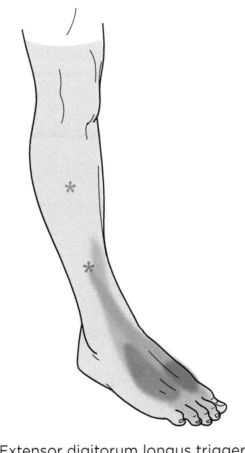

● Extensor digitorum longus trigger points
● Extensor hallucis longus trigger points

Ankle/Toe Extensors
Extensor Digitorum Longus, Extensor Hallucis Longus

Where it hurts: Deep pain on the part of the top of the foot that goes over the toes.

You might also be experiencing: Weakness and cramping on the top of the foot at night.

It's often caused by: Tripping and falling, stubbing your toe, activities that involve kicking a ball or using pedals.

Step 1: Treat the Spine

- Using the Big Bend Backnobber or a similar tool, apply pressure to the paraspinal muscles in the deep lower back, right next to vertebrae L4–S1.

Step 2: Floss the Nerve

- Perform the Sitting Toe Pointer nerve floss (page 159).

Step 3: Treat the Trigger Points

- Try to point your toes (if this area is really tight, you might not be able to). You'll feel a pull where one or more of these muscles are shortened, about two to three fingers' width to the outside of the shinbone.

- Find the tender area where you felt the pull. Fingers or a Thumbby work here, but my favorite tool is the Tiger Tail.

- Hold the pressure for between 10 and 90 seconds per tender spot.

Step 4: Gently Move

- Sit in a chair in a neutral position with your treatment leg out in front of you, knee straight or slightly bent, heel resting on the floor.

- To lengthen the muscle, exhale as you slowly flex the treatment ankle so that your toes point up toward your nose. Then let the ankle relax.

- To shorten the muscle, exhale as you slowly extend the treatment ankle, pointing your toes forward toward the floor. Then let the ankle relax again.

- Repeat a total of five times.

Other muscles to treat: The tibialis anterior (page 168) and peroneus muscles (page 166).

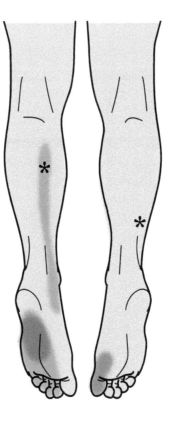

● Flexor digitorum longus trigger points
● Flexor hallucis longus trigger points

Ankle/Toe Flexors
Flexor Digitorum Longus, Flexor Hallucis Longus

Where it hurts: The bottom of the foot in front of the heel, behind the ball of the foot, and the big toe and its ball.

You might also be experiencing: Pain when you walk, hammertoes, or "claw toes."

It's often caused by: Walking or jogging on uneven surfaces like trails and beaches.

Step 1: **Treat the Spine**

- Using the Big Bend Backnobber or a similar tool, apply pressure to the paraspinal muscles in the deep lower back, right next to vertebrae L5–S2.

Step 2: **Floss the Nerve**

- Perform the Sitting Toe Pointer nerve floss (page 159).

Step 3: **Treat the Trigger Points**

- Cross your treatment ankle over the opposite knee. The tender region is just behind the tibia, or shinbone.

- Press between the bone and the overlying gastrocnemius (page 162) and soleus (page 164) muscles with either of your thumbs. Go down and then roll under the bone. (No tool can do this.)

- Press from back to front behind the lower third of the bone on the outside of your leg.

- Hold the pressure for between 10 and 90 seconds per tender spot.

Step 4: **Gently Move**

- Sit in a chair in a neutral position with your treatment leg out in front of you, knee straight or slightly bent, heel resting on the floor.

- To lengthen the muscle, exhale as you slowly flex the treatment ankle so that your toes point up toward your nose. Then let the ankle relax.

- To shorten the muscle, exhale as you slowly extend the treatment ankle, pointing your toes forward toward the floor. Then let the ankle relax again.

- Repeat a total of five times.

Other muscles to treat: The gastrocnemius (page 162), tibialis anterior (page 168), or intrinsic foot muscles (pages 176 and 178).

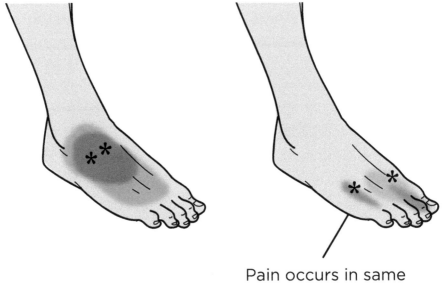

Pain occurs in same location on bottom of foot.

● Extensor digitorum brevis and extensor hallucis brevis trigger points
● Interosseus muscles trigger points.

Dorsal Foot Muscles
Extensor Digitorum Brevis, Extensor Hallucis Brevis, Interosseous Muscles

Where it hurts: On top of the foot and into the toes.

You might also be experiencing: N/A

It's often caused by: Tight shoes.

Step 1: Treat the Spine

- Using the Big Bend Backnobber or a similar tool, apply pressure to the paraspinal muscles in the deep lower back, right next to vertebrae L5–S1.

Step 2: Floss the Nerve

- Perform the Sitting Toe Pointer nerve floss (page 159).

Step 3: Treat the Trigger Points

- Press on the top of the foot to find trigger points in the superficial muscles. Use a Thumbby or trap it with your Acumasseur, though a finger works in a pinch.

- You can treat the deeper interossei (that's a fancy way of saying "between the bones") by gently pushing the relevant bone up from under the foot, exposing the muscle on the side so you can apply pressure.

- Hold the pressure for between 10 and 90 seconds per tender spot.

Step 4: Gently Move

- Sit in a chair in a neutral position with your treatment leg out in front of you, knee straight or slightly bent, heel resting on the floor.

- To lengthen the muscle, exhale as you slowly extend the treatment ankle, keeping your heel in place as you point your toes forward toward the floor. Then let the ankle relax.

- To shorten the muscle, exhale as you slowly flex the treatment foot so that your toes point up toward your nose. Then let the ankle relax again.

- Repeat a total of five times.

Other muscles to treat: The plantar foot muscles (page 178). Sometimes it's worthwhile to treat all the foot muscles—it doesn't take long.

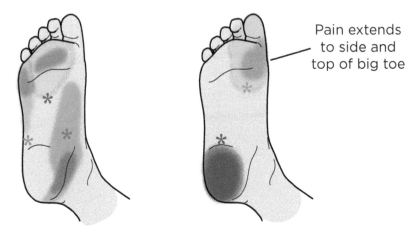

Pain extends to side and top of big toe

- Abductor digiti minimi trigger points
- Flexor digitorum brevis trigger points
- Abductor hallucis trigger points
- Quadratus plantae trigger points
- Flexor hallucis brevis trigger points

Plantar Foot Muscles
Abductor Hallucis, Abductor Digiti Minimi, Flexor Digitorum Brevis, Quadratus Plantae, Flexor Hallucis Brevis

Where it hurts: The bottom of the feet.

You might also be experiencing: Numbness and/or tingling.

It's often caused by: Old shoes, flat feet, and excessive rolling of the foot when it hits the ground. It can even be caused by a long second toe.

Step 1: **Treat the Spine**
- Using the Big Bend Backnobber or a similar tool, apply pressure to the paraspinal muscles in the deep lower back, right next to vertebrae L5–S3.

Step 2: **Floss the Nerve**

- Do the Sitting Toe Pointer nerve floss (page 159) and/or the Lean and Look nerve floss (page 158).

Step 3: **Treat the Trigger Points**

- First, pull the big toe back slightly. Move it up and down, feeling for movement between its base and the inside bottom of the foot, or between its base and the lower middle of the foot.

- Search along the movement areas for tender spots to press.

- Use a Thumbby to press on the tender spots, holding the pressure for 10 to 90 seconds per spot.

- Now pull the other four toes back as a group, feeling for movement just under the ball of the foot. Locate and press any tender spots in that area for 10 to 90 seconds each.

- Pull the four smaller toes back as a group again. This time, feel for movement just in front of the heel, and seek out tender spots on both sides of the band that you find. Apply and hold pressure for 10 to 90 seconds per tender spot.

- There can be a lot of tender areas, but be persistent—it pays off!

Step 4: **Gently Move**

- Sit in a chair in a neutral position with your treatment leg out in front of you, knee straight or slightly bent, heel resting on the floor.

- To lengthen the muscle, exhale as you slowly extend the treatment ankle, keeping your heel in place as you point your toes forward toward the floor. Then let the ankle relax.

- To shorten the muscle, exhale as you slowly flex the treatment foot so that your toes point up toward your nose. Then let the ankle relax again.

- Repeat a total of five times.

Other muscles to treat: The gastrocnemius (page 162) and the tibialis posterior (page 170).

Resources

Where to Order Tools

PressurePositive.com for the Big Bend Backnobber and the Knobble
TheOriginalWorm.com for the Original Worm
TigerTailUSA.com for the Tiger Tail
Amazon.com for the Thumbby
DermCreations.com for O$_2$ Derm Relief Gel

Find a Trigger Point Therapist

The very first choice should be accredited members of the National Association of Myofascial Trigger Point Therapists, which you can find at **https://www.myofascialtherapy.org/find-a-therapist**.

You can also consult the Neuromuscular Therapy Center's practitioner directory at **https://nmtcenter.com/practitioner-directory**.

Books

The Trigger Point Therapy Workbook by Clair Davies and Amber Davies

Healing through Trigger Point Therapy by Devin J. Starlanyl and John Sharkey

Trigger Point Therapy for Low Back Pain by Mary Biancalana and Sharon Sauer

Travell, Simons & Simons' Myofascial Pain and Dysfunction: The Trigger Point Manual by Joseph M. Donnelly, et al.

References

Calvert, Robert Noah. "Pages from History: Swedish Massage." *Massage Magazine*, April 24, 2014.

Gilbert, Christopher. "Better Chemistry through Breathing: The Story of Carbon Dioxide and How It Can Go Wrong." *Biofeedback* 33, no. 3 (Fall 2005): 100–104.

Gilbert, Christopher. "Hyperventilation and the Body." *Accident and Emergency Nursing* 7, no. 3 (July 1999): 130–140. doi:10.1016/s0965-2302 (99)80072-1.

Lerner, Barron H. "A Nurse Gains Fame in the Days of Polio." *New York Times*. December 26, 2013. https://well.blogs.nytimes.com/2013/12/26/a-nurse-gains-fame-in-the-days-of-polio/.

Sella, Gabriel and Richard Finn. *Myofascial Pain Syndrome: Manual Trigger Point & S-EMG Biofeedback Therapy Methods*. Gen Med Publishing, 2001.

Shah, Jay and Elizabeth A. Gilliams. "Uncovering the Biochemical Milieu of Myofascial Trigger Points Using in vivo Microdialysis: An Application of Muscle Pain Concepts to Myofascial Pain Syndrome." *Journal of Bodywork and Movement Therapies* 12, no. 4 (October 2008): 371–384. doi:10.1016/j.jbmt.2008.06.006.

Simons, David G. "Orphan Organ." *Journal of Musculoskeletal Pain* 15, no. 2 (2007): 7–9. doi:10.1300/J094v15n02_03.

Taylor, George. *An Exposition of the Swedish Movement-Cure: Embracing the History and Philosophy of This System of Medical Treatment, With Examples of Single Movements, and Directions for Their Use in Various Forms of Chronic Disease, Forming a Complete Manual of Exercises*. New York: Fowler and Wells Publishers, 1860.

Travell, Janet and David G. Simons. *Myofascial Pain and Dysfunction: The Trigger Point Manual*. Williams and Wilkins, 1983.

Index

Symptom Index

heel, 164–165

instep, 166–167, 168–169

toes, 176–177

top of foot, 172–173, 176–177

Front of body pain, 112–113

Frozen shoulder, 70–71

Full-body tightness, 34–35

G

Grasping difficulty, 94–95

Groin pain, 130–131, 152–153

H

Hammertoes, 174–175

Hamstrings don't release, 150–151

Hand pain

back of hand, 72–73, 94–95

fingers, 92–93, 94–95, 98–99

fleshy area between thumb and index
finger, 86–87, 88–89

palm of hand, 94–95, 96–97

thumbs, 82–83, 100–101,
102–103

Head pain, 34–35, 50–51

back of head, 44–45

forehead, 38–39, 44–45, 50–51

scalp, 44–45

temple, 36–37, 56–58

Headaches, 56–58

Heartburn, 128–129, 130–131

Heel pain, 164–165

Hip pain, 126–127, 136–137, 148–149

Hunched shoulders, 56–58

I

Inability to stand straight
at waist, 140–141

J

Jaw pain, 36–37, 38–39, 40–41, 42–
43, 56–58

K

Knee pain, 154–156

back of knee, 162–163

front of knee, 138–139

inner sides, 142–143

outer sides, 142–143

Knees, inability to move outward, 152–153

L

Leg pain, 152–153

down back of leg, 144–145

down back of thigh, 148–149

inner thigh, 142–143, 150–151, 152–153

outer thigh, 136–137, 142–143

side of leg, 144–145

upper back of thigh, 154–156

upper front of thigh, 140–141

Legs can't separate, 150–151

Locking knees, 142–143

M

Mouth pain

teeth pain, 42–43

teeth sensitivity, 36–37

tightness when opening
mouth wide, 38–39

N

Nausea, 128–129

Neck pain

crook of neck, 54–55, 56–58

difficulty turning neck, 54–55, 80–81

up side of neck, 56–58

Numbness, 178–179

Numbness down the arms, 52–53,
116–117

Numbness in back of arm, 84–85

Numbness on outside of thigh, 136–137

P

Pain when leaning back, 124–125

Pain when using hands to press
down, 119–121

Pain when using stairs, 164–165

Pain while turning side to side, 112–113

Muscle Index

Acknowledgments

There are way too many people to list in this brief section who have helped prepare me to write this book in many ways. The first is my wife, Carol. There would be no book if she hadn't made sure I had the time, quiet, and encouragement to keep writing. She put me through trigger point school, worked beside me in many settings, and gently, graciously took this path with me. She is also a talented therapist and has spent many years pushing me to "keep it simple."

My daughter, Sarah, has been a model for my pictures, a test subject for new techniques, my photographer, my videographer, and an all-around good sport for putting up with a dad who was always at work.

My editor, Lauren O'Neal, has been simply amazing. She has been by my side with encouragement, pointed questions, answers to my many questions, amazing ideas, and gentle nudging. There could be no book without her.

I've had some amazing mentors in my journey of learning about pain and trigger points, and I've been supported by the students, faculty, donors, and board of the Pittsburgh School of Pain Management, where I was kept off the street for 18 years of my life. The things we did together were amazing. Their support through thick and thin allowed me to actually become an instructor.

I never would have made it through my initial schooling without the incredible support of Providence Orthodox Presbyterian Church in Denver. They supported me even though I was on the other side of the country, and they were there for me when I returned.

Of course, the things I've said poorly or left out are my own responsibility. I am first and foremost a man who makes mistakes. I hope you find help in these pages. That's really why I wanted to write it. I really hate pain.

About the Author

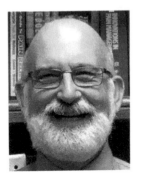

Richard Finn, LMT, CMTPT, is a graduate of Trinity College of the Bible with a degree in Biblical counseling, the Academy of Myotherapy and Physical Fitness, and the Academy of Health Sciences (Fort Sam Houston USAR, physical therapy specialist). He earned his CMT through the Life Credit Program at the Colorado School of Healing Arts. He is a board-certified member of the National Association of Myofascial Trigger Point Therapists and served as president from 1992 to 1994. Richard has served on the board of advisors of the Fibromyalgia Research Foundation and on the executive committee of the National Association of Myofascial Trigger Point Therapists. He has coauthored a set of wall charts of muscle length tests with C. M. Shifflett and a textbook, *Myofascial Pain Syndrome: Manual Trigger Point & S-EMG Biofeedback Therapy Methods*, with Gabriel Sella, MD. He demonstrates myofascial trigger point treatment on his YouTube channel at ChristianPainManagement.com.